Looking for the Bigger Picture in General Practice

This thought-provoking book exposes and challenges the hidden assumptions of modern medicine: the body is a kind of machine, symptoms must be caused by disease, health depends on healthcare, prevention is better than cure, things that can be measured are more real than those that cannot, how we see things is how they are, relationships are peripheral to medical care, and proper doctors just keep going. It encourages readers to reconsider how they think about health and the wider healthcare system, and how to look after patients, themselves and each other as clinicians.

Recognising that many of the problems in the NHS and other healthcare systems are complex and not just due to overwhelming demand or staff shortage, the pieces of writing in this collection draw attention to the gap between our understanding of these issues and our everyday experience. Using vivid analogies and colourful characters, the author invites readers to fit the pieces together and look at the bigger picture that emerges.

This book is intended as a tonic for clinically active GPs in training and beyond who deal with the consequences of small-picture thinking on a daily basis. It will also be of interest to GP trainers, including course organisers and those involved in curriculum development, and other primary care health professionals and administrators.

Ben Hoban has been a GP at Wonford Green Surgery in Exeter since 2001. He is a GP trainer, appraiser, and mentor, and the winner of the 2025 Kieran Sweeney Prize for medical writing.

Looking for the Bigger Picture in General Practice

Assorted Reflections

Ben Hoban

CRC Press
Taylor & Francis Group
Boca Raton London New York

CRC Press is an imprint of the
Taylor & Francis Group, an **informa** business

Designed cover image: Getty Images. Credit: Colin McDonald.

First edition published 2026
by CRC Press
2385 NW Executive Center Drive, Suite 320, Boca Raton FL 33431

and by CRC Press
4 Park Square, Milton Park, Abingdon, Oxon, OX14 4RN

CRC Press is an imprint of Taylor & Francis Group, LLC

© 2026 Ben Hoban

The material in this book began life as articles for the Life and Times section of the *British Journal of General Practice* or for the *BJGPLife* website and is adapted with permission.

ISBN: 978-1-041-09844-7 (hbk)
ISBN: 978-1-041-09839-3 (pbk)
ISBN: 978-1-003-65204-5 (ebk)

DOI: 10.1201/9781003652045

Typeset in Sabon
by SPi Technologies India Pvt Ltd (Straive)

For Abi

Contents

Foreword

Next to my bedside, I have two things: a pile of books, and a pen and paper. When I wake in the middle of the night, I can jot down the thoughts that stop me going back to sleep. In a GP career spent "looking for the bigger picture," this is just how I do that. This volume by Ben Hoban is a welcome addition to my creative pile.

Even as a child, I always had a pile of books. What has changed over a professional lifetime is the addition of pen and paper. I have learned that the wisdom of general practice is defined not simply by the things we glean from reading books; but rather by how we use what we know to make a difference for people, practice and communities. Our wisdom comes not just from gathering knowledge, but from the ability to use what we gather, critically and creatively, to originate new knowledge-in-context. For me, that process often starts with the reflections that appear on my bedside notepad.

"But I haven't got time for this, just tell me the key action points." These are the words I have often heard during a career spent seeking to challenge and change how people understand the bigger picture. In an era of Clinical Knowledge Summaries that tell us what to do, I am often asked what use reflection is? Ben's writing provides a powerful response, by making visible the deep critical reflective thinking that defines the knowledge work of our professional wisdom.

So how did I listen to Ben? I simply dived in: with curiosity, no expectations, no boxes to tick, no 'fixed learning outcomes.' My bedside notepaper records 'permission to be curious.' In 'Seeing the tiger,' Ben reminds us that "noticing" is part of our job as doctors. It's a first step to help us understand and so explain, because explanations help patients "experience [symptoms] differently and so start to feel better." How often has the work of explaining helped me to feel better too?

Later I explore 'Scientists after all' and read that "The scientific method has traditionally been about three things: empiricism, reductionism and generalisation." Now my sleep is disturbed! I start with bookish thoughts about the scientific practices that don't fit that framework. But quickly I move on to thinking about the many practising GPs and trainees I have met over the years for whom science (and so evidence) is still synonymous with reductionism – especially those who ask me for 'action points.' So, what this chapter triggers for me are reflections on why professional views of science exist and persist, and crucially, how we creatively challenge them.

For me, this book is a "hand on the swing"[1] for our profession. It is the gentle push that gives us the "confidence to start moving again," reclaiming our independent professional thinking. For it is not what we know, but how we use what we know, that defines our professional practice. So, this book, along with the reflective exercises it invites and enables, will become a core text for our work in WiseGP to support GPs to hone their professional skills. Wherever your reflective space is, I encourage you to keep this book nearby.

To quote Ben, "General Practice is ... cutting edge, and we shouldn't be afraid to own it." This book can help you do just that.

Joanne Reeve
FRCGP, Professor of Primary Care,
Hull, York Medical School,
Founder of WiseGP

Note

1 Falling off the swing.

Introduction

Something strange is afoot in UK general practice. Surgeries and health centres are providing more appointments than ever before, but patients still struggle to see their doctor. At a time when the benefits of personally continuous medical care are firmly established, we are adopting ways of working that seem designed instead to fragment care. Despite being in many ways far healthier than previous generations, we feel less confident in our health. Our thinking lets us down and so we build machines to think for us, but they have not made us wise. These things are parts of a puzzle: in order to make sense of them, it is not enough simply to hold each one up to the light; we must rather fit the pieces together, stand back, and look at the bigger picture that emerges.

Modern western medicine represents a phenomenally successful way of doing exactly the opposite. As an essentially scientific project, it is based on the idea that the whole is best understood by breaking it down into anonymous parts; it is more interested in the body in general than in anybody in particular, and in diseases rather than the people affected by them. No matter how much we stand to gain from such an approach, it is predictable that it will have its limits. We can measure precisely someone's blood pressure, the concentration of sodium in their bodily fluids, or the diameter of their common bile duct without learning anything meaningful about them, just as we can excise a tumour from their body without necessarily doing them any good. It would be wrong to fault medicine for not being something else, but the reality is that we routinely overlook its shortcomings. We have privileged a limited scientific approach at the expense of others capable of balancing it because we are beguiled by details and clarity, and the bigger picture can be messy.

This preference for tidiness in our thinking has given rise to what Michel Foucault called "the medical gaze," a commitment to seeing things from a narrowly biomedical perspective, and in highly concrete terms.[1] Under the medical gaze, there are many things that seem obvious: the body is a kind of machine whose parts break down and need to be fixed; symptoms are due to disease; what is measurable is more real than what is not; prevention is better than cure; and patients are best looked after by a practitioner with the necessary skills to deal with their presenting problem. All these statements are largely true, but not entirely, and not always; they are approximations, rational but impersonal, although we often take them at face value. Each involves the temporary suspension of someone's humanity, the transformation of a person into a patient and of individuals into data points within a population, and as with all temporary measures, our memory of what preceded them soon fades.

It is the tragedy of contemporary healthcare systems that, as a result of this outlook, they focus less on enabling whole people to live healthy and meaningful lives and more on fixing or maintaining diseased body parts and preventing disease in the rest. It is unsurprising that within this environment general practice, with its emphasis on individual people and their stories and concerns, has become neglected and misunderstood. Some may protest that any impersonal tendencies within the health service are glitches and anomalies, when the reality is perhaps the opposite: it is a dehumanising system which is only made tolerable through the kindness and common sense of those working in and using it. The solution is certainly not to mandate more kindness or common sense, but we might reasonably ask how we have ended up with a system so lacking in both to start with.

Frustration of one kind or another is the constant companion of anyone working in the National Health Service, and in the daily rush to complete tasks and meet targets it is often simpler to go with the flow than to ponder these things. We have become adept at managing this dysfunction, keeping our heads down to deal with the details in front of us, and rarely taking a step back to look at the bigger picture which they make up, and which might place them in their proper context.

I hope that you find what follows both interesting and thought-provoking, but also that it will serve as a reminder of what is possible in general practice. It is easy to wear ourselves out doing work that is both unsatisfying and of limited benefit to patients. There are many factors contributing to this that are outside of our control, but by looking for a bigger picture in our thinking, our systems, our consultations and our practices, we may still find a way of working that is less draining, more satisfying, and of greater benefit to those we try to help.

All the pieces in this book were originally published in the *British Journal of General Practice* or online at BJGPLife.com between 2022 and 2025, although I have revised many of them since. Despite sharing various themes, they are intended to stand alone, and their loose organisation into four parts isn't to suggest that they should be read in any particular order, but rather to help the reader dip in and out according to their fancy at the time. I have written as a doctor with his colleagues in mind, although the writing should be accessible to anyone with an interest in healthcare.

I would like to thank Ed Fitzherbert, who first encouraged me to start writing for a wider audience; Andrew Papanikitas at the *BJGP*, who encouraged me to keep going and consider putting what I had written into a book; Joanne Reeve, for her kindness in writing the foreword; and Jo Koster at Taylor & Francis, who made it all happen. I would also like to thank my wife Abi, without whose support and knack for asking the right questions none of this would have been possible.

Reference

1. Foucault Michel, *The Birth of the Clinic: An Archaeology of Medical Perception*, Vintage Books, New York, 1963.

PART I

How We Think about Things

The European Reformation and the Age of Enlightenment that followed it may have freed us from our dependence on authority and tradition as sources of knowledge. By putting the focus on our ability to observe and understand the world for ourselves, though, they also forced us to confront the many errors inherent in both these processes. It is convenient to trust that when we open our eyes, we simply see things as they are, just as we simply listen to our patients and work out what is wrong with them. What actually happens is more complicated, however. At the level of our perception, our thinking and the stories we tell ourselves to make sense of life, as much depends on us as on the world, or the patient, in front of us.

What we see, hear and feel is certainly based on reality, although more loosely than it seems at the time. We do not perceive anything just because it is there, but because it corresponds with something that is also in our mind. Although reality is a continuous, complex whole, our ability to engage with it requires us to break it down into more manageable chunks which we can name and encode. It therefore feels easier to deal with nouns than verbs, and with numbers rather than narrative. We recognise what we know and expect, and pass over what we cannot make sense of. Our expectations vary from one situation to another, making the process strongly context-dependent, even though most of the time we are blissfully unaware of it.

Our thinking and decision-making also largely take place within a black box, driven by shortcuts and rules of thumb that we might deny if they were pointed out to us, and yet without which we would be forced to process our experience at the speed of a pocket calculator rather than a

DOI: 10.1201/9781003652045-1

super-computer. We think fast, and the price we pay is that we are prone to biases in our thinking which we cannot avoid. Even when we limit ourselves to making concrete diagnoses, we regularly get things wrong, not necessarily from a lack of time or knowledge, but because reality tends to be less concrete than we would like. It can be difficult to reserve judgement and uncomfortable to keep our minds open for long, and yet uncertainty is not always a veil which can be lifted in order to reveal the truth behind it, but rather a fog out of which a story takes shape one way or another under different conditions.

What should we do then, in such an uncertain world, where the stakes are high, and clear thinking can literally be a matter of life and death? We cannot simply try harder or practise more cautiously, nor can we bear such a heavy burden of responsibility alone. Most decisions that we make in good faith and in collaboration with our patients will be reasonable at the time, even if events subsequently prove them wrong, and learning to say sorry is a part of the process too. Perhaps we can make our way through the fog most successfully by recognising first that our thinking is necessarily fallible; then by considering what form our errors might take so that we can notice them more easily; and, finally, by acquiring a set of tools that meet the particular needs of general practice, even if we have to imagine them first.

Naming

Naming is always a significant act, conferring on its object both identity and status. A baby is recognised as both a new individual and a member of their family; medical students graduate from being known by a first name to using their new professional title; and an acute respiratory infection becomes a byword for death, disruption and misery of all kinds. There is often a choice of names – COVID-19 rather than Wuhan 'flu, for example – and in choosing, we necessarily also decide how to view a thing, and how to relate to it.

To name something is to define it: literally, to fix an end or limit to what it might be; to make it a known and finite quantity. Naming allows us to grasp something, to comprehend and contain it as one might apprehend and detain a thief. There is a long tradition in folklore and fiction of the *true name*, which is not just a handle of convenience for a thing, but somehow expresses its essence or hidden self, allowing it to be controlled by one who is in the know. The literary applications are generally in the realm of magic, but it's easy to see the same idea in medicine. A person's true name is now their genetic code, which can be read and re-written to change their nature, and simply mentioning *DNA* is enough to evoke this, even if most people have a limited understanding of deoxyribonucleic acid: chemicals have names too. Patients may recognise a medicine's brand name, but doctors know another, harder to pronounce and written in smaller print on the box, which allows them to prescribe it. In fact, a large part of what we do is directed towards discovering the secret names of illnesses so that we can master them. Many conditions are either benign or self-limiting, and there are remedies available to treat their symptoms, but others lurk in the shadows, gathering their strength until they are ready to emerge and overwhelm us: we must recognise their traces and name them first.

DOI: 10.1201/9781003652045-2

What if we pick the wrong name, though? The question of diagnosis leads inevitably to that of misdiagnosis, which may be worse than none at all. Although naming something tells us what it is and how to deal with it, such clarity comes at a cost, in that we assume we have fully understood the situation and no longer look for nuances or alternative explanations. Consider too that we can only choose a name from among those that readily come to mind in a given situation: what if there is a bigger picture which we can't yet see? The name easily becomes a smooth stone fitting comfortably into the palm of our hand, which we hold onto even after new information presents itself. Sometimes we would do better to throw it away: the tendency to close our minds prematurely is a recognised cause of medical error.[1]

Naming a patient's suffering can be therapeutic, acknowledging it as real and setting boundaries around it. It can also be problematic, inasmuch as all diagnoses are generic, while a patient's experience is unique to them; the name may be accurate, but only gives us the illusion of understanding. When a patient feels overwhelmed by what they're going through, it may be enough just to acknowledge this, without trying to persuade them that there is a limit to what feels limitless, or that by implication, it's not as bad as it seems.

There are therefore both advantages and disadvantages in giving something a name, and a tension between our need to diagnose promptly and accurately, and to recognise the individual variations of different illnesses as well as their common patterns. If naming demonstrates our mastery over disease and allows us to end the consultation and call our next patient, it seems likely that we will generally be biased in favour of making a diagnosis. Perhaps it would be better, though, to cultivate a little less certainty, to reserve judgement and keep our diagnoses provisional where possible. We can still acknowledge and validate someone's suffering on its own terms, while being open about the uncertainty that is inherent in medicine and involving them in deciding what to do about it, rather than reaching for an off-the-shelf management plan. We can call this being "patient-centred" if we choose, but perhaps it would be better not to give it a name: after all, should there really be any other centre to someone's care?

Reference

1. Croskerry P. The Importance of Diagnostic Errors in Diagnosis and Strategies to Minimize Them. *Acad Med* 2003;78:775–780.

Learning to Live with Cognitive Bias*

You're probably familiar with the idea of cognitive bias, our minds' tendency to play tricks on us; little acts of sabotage perpetrated by the gremlins in our head that stop us from seeing what's right in front of us and trip us up as we go about the business of diagnosing and treating patients. Just as traditional folklore contains a whole menagerie of such supernatural mischief-makers, there is also a well-stocked zoo of different biases, from the mundanely-named base-rate neglect and the gambler's fallacy, to the more colourful Pollyanna principle,[1, 2] and wandering among its enclosures for any length of time may make us question how much we ever get right. Of course, if you're prone to *exceptionalism*, you might just smile and shake your head at how easily other people get in a muddle.

As a concept, cognitive bias is linked with the idea that we have two complementary ways of thinking.[3, 4] What we usually understand as thinking – consciously processing information step-by-step – turns out to be painfully slow. It can only handle small sets of data, and only if they're readily available, limiting its usefulness. The other kind of thinking is far more powerful, integrating huge datasets from multiple sources below our level of conscious awareness, including distant memories and subtle environmental cues. It is so fast and distinct from its slower cousin that we don't even consider it thought, referring to it instead as intuition, gut-feeling or "acting-in-the-moment." Its weakness, though, is that it is prone to cognitive bias. To some extent, we can of course recognise this and make allowances for it. The tendency to bias in our fast thinking, however, is so fundamental that it actually demonstrates a much bigger truth.

* An earlier version of this piece was published as: Hoban B. Learning to live with cognitive bias, *Br J Gen Pract*. 2022 Sep, doi: 10.3399/bjgp22X720581.

DOI: 10.1201/9781003652045-3

Fast thinking relies on heuristics, cognitive short-cuts and rules of thumb that work by association and extrapolation to bridge our mental gaps and fill in the blanks. We rely on these heuristics not just in our thinking, but in our day-to-day experience of reality. We all have a literal blind spot in our visual field, of which we're so unaware that identifying it feels like a party trick.[5] Similarly, although the perception of colour is limited to the very centre of our visual fields, there is no point beyond which we suddenly experience our surroundings in black-and-white. *Cognitive blindness* prevents us from seeing something unexpected even when it stands in front of us and waves.[6] In each of these cases, we are integrating incoming sensory data with extensive background knowledge of how things usually work to make sense of the world around us. We do this so smoothly that we don't even realise: we think we're simply observing reality, when in fact what we see depends at least partly on what our brain tells us to see. The same process affects our perception and reasoning during the consultation, so that we notice most easily whatever conforms to our expectations, think first of what is familiar to us, and downplay the significance of anything that gets in the way. It's not just that we commit errors: our entire mental operating system is built in such a way that they are inevitable.

Can we ever hope to see things clearly, then, or are we doomed instead to suffer at the hands of these mischievous sprites that curdle our diagnostic milk, and the will-o'-the-wisps that lead us astray? The path that winds through the mire of symptoms, signs and special investigations is treacherous at the best of times, and the only way to keep our feet dry is not to walk it. A pair of waders is a sensible precaution, then, no matter how confident we are in our clinical skills; as we say goodbye to our patients, we might do better to ask ourselves how we might have got things wrong than to congratulate ourselves on a good diagnosis or simply hope for the best. Indeed, being open about our propensity to error with ourselves, our patients and our colleagues makes it easier to learn from experience when something goes wrong, as it inevitably does on occasion. Patients tend to value doctors who are fallible but willing to help them through life's difficulties by embracing their own part in the drama, as one person with another, rather than pursuing some false vision of detached objectivity. We will never be free from bias or error. Our security lies not in perfection, but in recognising and learning from our imperfections.

References

1. Croskery P. The Importance of Cognitive Errors in Diagnosis and Strategies to Minimize Them. *Acad Med* 2003;78:775–780.

2. Pohl R., ed. *Cognitive Illusions: Intriguing Phenomena in Judgement, Thinking and Memory*, 2nd edition, Psychology Press, London, 2016.

3. Kahneman Daniel, *Thinking, Fast, Slow*, Penguin, New York, 2012.

4. Lehrer Jonah, *The Decisive Moment: How the Brain Makes up Its Mind*, Canongate Books Ltd, Edinburgh, 2010.

5. http://webmd.com/eye-health/eye-blind-spot

6. http://youtube.com/watch?v=vJG698U2Mvo

Making It Real

The world that you see every day when you wake up and open your eyes is not real. What you experience when you look out of the window and finish your cup of tea, when you travel to work and when you call your first patient is a simulation, extrapolated from limited sensory data and based on a model in your head which you have spent your whole life developing. The reason we don't realise this is that it's a very good simulation, and it's all we have.[1,2]

If that seems strange, consider what happens when you are dreaming or lost in a book, remembering your last holiday or planning the next one: you see, hear and feel things that are not happening, often with an undeniable sense of reality. Is it such a leap to imagine that our day-to-day experiences arises in a similar way?

We can look at a degraded image of something familiar and see only black-and-white splodges, but once we know what we are looking at, we cannot unsee what they represent.[3] Patterns of light and shade falling on our retina are the starting point, but our perception is driven by the mental constructs we associate with these patterns, by *recognition*. The image encodes the experience, as do words on a page, but the two are not the same. We look at the world, but we see what our brain tells us to see.

Think about how easy it is to recognise faces in inanimate objects: we understand that things are not people, but sometimes we can't help reacting momentarily as if they were.[4] We project the construct *smile* onto the barest suggestion of a sagging horizontal line with two dots above it, in the same way that a social media filter projects a stylised construct of a face onto the outline it recognises in our photo.

This also applies to our awareness of our own body and mind: there is a sensory substrate which informs what we feel, but does not determine it.

DOI: 10.1201/9781003652045-4

We are sensitive to the concentration of glucose in our bloodstream, but we never actually *feel* it directly, in the same way that we don't *feel* excitement or fear when the vehicle we're in accelerates into a steep drop. Instead, our brains project these impressions onto ambiguous signals from our bodies, based on contextual factors like whether it's lunchtime or not, and whether we're on a rollercoaster or an icy road in the fog.[5] At other times, we feel nothing at all: the grandfather clock in the hall is still ticking but we stopped hearing it some time ago.

What all of this comes down to is that we have no way of experiencing reality directly; we only see, hear and feel our interpretation of that reality, without ever realising that there is a difference.

My father wrote that "Reality is ungraspable. For convenience we use a limited-reality consensus in which work can be done, transport arranged and essential services provided. The *real* reality is something else."[6] As doctors, we tend to recognise this in special cases like phantom limb pain and hallucinations, but most of the time we behave as if the reality and the limited-reality consensus, our mental model, were the same thing: symptoms are either due to disease, or the patient is imagining them or making them up. When someone asks you whether you're telling them it's all in their head, the most accurate answer is: *Yes, but isn't everything?*

A large part of our work as General Practitioners consists of managing the space between the model and the reality, the gap behind the sofa cushions of the world in which we find not loose change and biscuit crumbs, but unexplained suffering, and hurt that seems to have no concrete origin but is inescapably real.

When patients describe their symptoms in vivid terms, it's not for the sake of drama: they are simply changing their experience into words. Someone having a heart attack actually feels the elephant sitting on their chest. The person with peripheral neuropathy doesn't feel a burning pain; *they feel their legs burning.* In these examples, there is an obvious incongruity between what someone feels and what they can see: there is no elephant, and the legs are not on fire. At other times, though, patients have no way of checking their senses: if you feel as though something terrible is happening inside your pelvis, how do you know that it isn't? When patients report sensations for which there appears to be no clear pathological cause, it is because their brain is simulating a reality that makes sense of incoming information from their body, based on the model in their head. In this respect, what they feel is qualitatively no different from any other sensation, regardless of whether there is a distinct physical cause or not. When a patient insists that they know their body, they are telling the truth, even though that truth may be more subtle than they realise.

It is our job as doctors to recognise the significance of what our patients tell us, and to help them understand and manage what is happening to them. This applies not just in cases where their symptoms are indicative of this or that disease, however, but also in those where it becomes apparent that there is no identifiable disease. In both scenarios, our job includes agreeing an explanation that makes sense to the patient, helping them to recalibrate their mental model and simulate more accurately what is happening to them. This is a delicate business, and heavily dependent on trust. If we want to go beyond the textbook drill of diagnosing, treating and calling the next patient, we need to think less about engaging our patients, and show them rather that they have successfully engaged us, that we have not just heard their symptoms, but felt the weight of them ourselves, and we must find a way of explaining their experience in terms that make sense to them, that makes what we say *real*.[7] If we can do this, we will help our patients not just to understand their symptoms differently, but potentially to experience them differently and to start to feel better.

References

1. Van den Bergh O, Witthöft M, Petersen S, Brown RJ. Symptoms and the Body: Taking the Inferential Leap. *Neurosci Biobehav Rev* 2017;74:185–203.

2. Henningsen P et al. On behalf of the EURONET-SOMA group, Persistent Physical Symptoms as Perceptual Dysregulation: A Neuropsychobehavioural Model and Its Clinical Implications. *Psychosom Med* 2018;80:422–431.

3. Example of a two-tone (aka 'Mooney') image (researchgate.net). http://research gate.net/figure/Example-of-a-two-tone-aka-Mooney-image-On-first-viewing-this-image-appears-as-a_fig4_326466342

4. For example: 26 Faces in Everyday Objects. http://boredpanda.com/objects-with-faces/?utm_source=bing&utm_medium=organic&utm_campaign=organic

5. Barrett Lisa Feldman, *How Emotions are Made: The Secret Life of the Brain*, Pan, New York, 2017.

6. Hoban Russell, *The Moment under the Moment*, Jonathan Cape, London, 1992.

7. Dowrick CF, Ring A, Humphris GM and Salmon P. Normalisation of Unexplained Symptoms by General Practitioners: A Functional Typology. *Br J Gen Pract*, 2004;54:165–170.

Telling a Good Story

We talk about taking a history from a patient in the same way as we talk about taking blood: collecting a medium from which clinically useful information about the individual can be extracted. Histories – stories – are not just about individual people or events, though, but about the significance we attribute to them: the *hero* and the *villain*; the *problem* and the *resolution*. You and I may observe the same event and give quite different accounts of it, based on our own understanding of what we've seen, which will, in turn, be influenced by how we felt at the time, our past experiences, and our personal norms and expectations. We may have the same information available to us, but telling a story involves context too, and deciding which details to include and how to connect them: it is an active process through which we make sense of our experience rather than simply registering it.[1, 2]

There are times, too, when the sense comes first, and the story establishes itself from the available elements. I may have a gut feeling that something is wrong, in which case you must be the villain, the others must be in on it, and I'd better do something about it right now.[3] The facts here are secondary: our naked impression clothes itself with whatever is to hand. This is arguably the basis for cognitive distortions such as fundamental attribution error and confirmation bias:[4] in a story, someone doing something bad must be *the bad guy*, and once the story starts to take shape, we can only assimilate new information in a way that fits the plot. The way to change the narrative in this situation is to alter the overall impression rather than arguing over the details.

Patients come to their appointments with an assortment of narrative elements: context, facts, interpretation and impression, in various stages of assembly. Our privilege in the consultation is to collaborate with them in

DOI: 10.1201/9781003652045-5

building these elements into a story – however limited – that makes sense. *I've caught a cold and it's gone to my chest. It's because I've been too busy with work to look after myself, but I know what to do now, and it should get better soon.*

By assigning a role in the narrative to each fact or circumstance, an effective story connects how things were, how they are now, and how they might be in the future; the more details it connects, the greater its explanatory power, and the more compelling it seems. Likewise, a story in which things happen for a reason, and big things happen for big reasons, feels inherently more believable. Conspiracy theories gain a following not because they are rational, but because they include these three crucial narrative elements.[5] Conversely, the problem with a lot of what we tell patients is that despite being true, it doesn't feel very believable. A patient suffering from severe chronic back pain knows that there's something seriously wrong, and saying it's just a mechanical problem won't cut the mustard. A narrative approach could be to explain that the pain is caused by a disastrous cascade of events in the musculoskeletal and nervous systems; that the body is trying to protect itself but, tragically, making things worse; and that it's no wonder every day is a struggle if they're having to fight against their own body just to get out of bed in the morning!

We tend to listen to what our patients tell us with an ear to what might be clinically relevant, either excluding or suggesting a particular diagnosis, and to regard the rest, by default, as incidental. We have been trained to hear disease narratives, familiar tales in which the villain is the pathology. To our patients, though, these tales are often less well-known: they are trying to tell us a story about their experience, while we are listening out for one from a textbook, and we easily end up at cross-purposes. This is at times unavoidable, and it would be negligent to miss a significant diagnosis for the sake of spinning a yarn. On the other hand, there are many consultations in which either the diagnosis is already clear, or it becomes apparent that there is no diagnosis that will fit the facts. In both cases we may serve our patients best by agreeing with them an appropriate narrative, which helps them to make sense of what is happening to them and decide what to do next. We won't always be able to guarantee a happy ending, but we should still do our best to tell a good story.

References

1. Greenhalgh Trisha and Hurwitz Brian, eds. *Narrative Based Medicine: Dialogue and Discourse in Clinical Practice*, BMJ Publishing Group, London, 1998.

2. Robertson Colin and Clegg Gareth, eds. *Storytelling in Medicine*, Routledge, Abingdon, 2016.

3. Barrett Lisa Feldman, *How Emotions Are Made: The Secret Life of the Brain*. Pan, New York, 2017.

4. Croskery P. The Importance of Cognitive Errors in Diagnosis and Strategies to Minimize Them. *Acad Med* 2003;78:775–780.

5. Brotherton Rob, *Suspicious Minds: Why we Believe Conspiracy Theories*. Bloomsbury Sigma, London, 2015.

Seeing the Tiger

General Practice may largely be a desk job, but every day at work we are surrounded by danger, and each trip to the waiting room to call the next patient, and every remote contact, is a walk to the well through tiger country. Most patients are not abusive, and burnout happens slowly and by degrees, but the risk of a serious missed diagnosis is always with us, like a predator's long shadow.

How we deal with clinical risk affects our usefulness as doctors, our efficiency in terms of the wider health service, and our own wellbeing. Patients seek reassurance, and yet we cannot give it absolutely. The longer we spend dotting the i's and crossing the t's with each patient, the more the waiting room fills up; the more uncertainty we swallow during the consultation, the more worry we take home with us in the evening. We readily accept the importance of knowing our stuff, getting on well with patients and working effectively with colleagues, but it can be difficult to know how to manage risk. Rather than practising either recklessly or defensively, however, we can mitigate a large part of this risk by taking note of a blind spot which we all share, a cognitive quirk that we neglect at our peril.

We generally reach a diagnosis in the same way as we pick out a familiar face from a crowd or make sense of words on a page: by recognising a pattern. In each case, a limited sensory input triggers the perception of a complete mental construct. We feel as if we're just seeing what's in front of us, when, in reality, we are generating a picture in our mind of what experience tells us we should be seeing, based on contextual cues.[1] This is a neat cognitive short-cut which allows us to interact with our environment in real time without having to work out from first principles what's

DOI: 10.1201/9781003652045-6

in front of us whenever we open our eyes. Its downside is that, just as we can read something without noticing the typos because we know what the words *ought to* look like, so we unconsciously edit the evidence of our own senses to increase the likelihood of recognition, filtering out anything incongruous.

This is the crux of our problem: in order to recognise something, we have to have an idea of what we're looking at, and having the wrong idea can mean that we don't see what is most important. Fortunately, we have a fail-safe mechanism to stop us getting this wrong. Just as recognising something involves matching a sensory picture with a mental one, *noticing* something is about detecting mismatches between the two. You probably won't be aware what colour socks your patient is wearing, but you'll notice if they're not a pair. Mismatches arise when the information we are trying to recognise is unfamiliar, unexpected or too ambiguous to fit any of the patterns in our database, and they produce a feeling of cognitive dissonance. This ought to prompt us to look at things differently until we find a better fit, just as toothache might prompt us to chew on the other side, but the danger is that we simply suppress it because it feels uncomfortable.

We may make sense of a moving pattern of vertical stripes by recognising it as a field of tall grass in the breeze. If we register a discrepancy between the visual input to our brain and the archive footage we associate with this phenomenon, we are immediately faced with a choice: do we reconsider what we're seeing or simply press on? We may have noticed the tiger, but chosen not to recognise it, without even realising.

If we want to avoid missing significant diagnoses, and tigers, we cannot examine every symptom or blade of grass exhaustively, but we can cultivate an openness to the sort of cognitive dissonance that points to unrecognised danger. If this is intuition,[2, 3] then there is certainly nothing magical about it. We need only regard our diagnoses as strictly provisional and ask ourselves: *What would something more serious look like, and how would I notice?* It is tempting to second-guess this through the routine use of investigations, but unless we have some sense of what we're looking for, the result may simply be false reassurance or incidental abnormalities. Being aware of our surroundings, letting our curiosity follow its nose, and allowing ourselves to tolerate a little ambiguity may be a more effective way of spotting tigers, and should make the walk to the well more enjoyable.[4]

References

1. Van den Bergh O, Witthöft M, Petersen S, Brown RJ. Symptoms and the Body: Taking the Inferential Leap. *Neurosci Biobehav Rev* 2017;74:185–203.

2. Friedemann Smith C, Drew S, Ziebland S, Nicholson B. Understanding the Role of GPs' Gut Feelings in Diagnosing Cancer in Primary Care: A Systematic Review and Meta-analysis of Existing Evidence. *Br J Gen Pract* 2020. https://doi.org/10.3399/bjgp20X712301

3. Greenhalgh T. Intuition and Evidence—Uneasy Bedfellows?. *Br J Gen Pract* 2002;52:395–400.

4. Hancock J, Mattick K. Tolerance of Ambiguity and Psychological Well-being in Medical Training: A Systematic Review. *Med Edu* 2020;54:125–137.

A Tyranny of Nouns*

You may not have considered this before, but doctors are inordinately fond of nouns. We keep and curate mental lists of them: the seven causes of a particular presentation or the key features of this or that disease. We think about patterns of illness as though they are concrete *things* with their own independent existence, although we'd struggle to put sepsis or depression into a pathology jar. We talk about the different aspects of ourselves – organs, limbs, emotions – in the same way: all nouns. We may tell one patient that their *bladder* has an *infection* which can be treated with *antibiotics*, and another that their *personality* has *mood instability* which can be treated with *anticonvulsants*, as if we were rearranging the flaps in a children's book to combine the astronaut's head with the lumberjack's trunk and the diver's legs. All of this may seem obvious and unremarkable, but it demonstrates the extent to which our thinking and our view of ourselves are influenced by reductionism: if we are no more than the sum of our parts, then in order for the whole to function well, we must simply fix the right part. How accurate is this really?

By and large, patients come to us not just with nouns, but with stories: these certainly include nouns but are driven along by verbs, words of action, backed up by adverbs, pronouns, and so on. Our professional ear filters these out or translates them into drier terms. *Yes, Mrs Jones, I understand that your lungs feel like they're full of treacle, but let's stick to the facts: a week of cough with sputum but no blood, you said. Any chest pain?* It's practical: you can see why German still capitalises its nouns.

* An earlier version of this piece was published as: Hoban B. A tyranny of nouns. *Br J Gen Pract*. 2023 Jan 26;73(727):79. doi: 10.3399/bjgp23X731925. PMID: 36702595; PMCID: PMC9888584.

DOI: 10.1201/9781003652045-7

On the odd occasion when patients lead with their nouns, it jars: *It's the pain, doc, it's making my anxiety worse.* Does this really tell us what we need to know? The instinctive response is to reach for more nouns: medication, therapy, a fit note. After a while it starts to feel just a little impersonal and repetitive, clichéd even. The reason is that nouns are good at communicating generic information, but not individual context. *Back pain secondary to overuse* is succinct but limited. A more meaningful way to express the same idea might be to suggest to someone that they've been overdoing it in the garden, and because their back isn't used to all the movement, the muscles are tensing up to try to protect it from injury.

There is also a danger that in talking about illness as a *thing*, we construe it as somehow foreign. *I have a pain in my foot* is a statement of location in the same way as *I have a stone in my shoe*, to which the obvious response is: get rid of it. By contrast, *My foot hurts* is a description of how a part of me is behaving, inviting the response: look after it. This is significant, in that virtually all the things that happen within the confines of our body are things that our body *does*. During an infection, fever, myalgia and all the other nouns on that particular list are simply the way our body responds to being invaded by a pathogen (yes, that one gets a noun). Even a gunshot rarely kills directly: it is our own body that pumps blood out of the wound, sucks air into it or triggers a pro-inflammatory cascade that makes it swell. The same applies to the mind. Consider the following statements which are semantically equivalent and see which feels most meaningful: *I have depression; I'm very sad; I feel as if I've lost something important to my sense of self.*

If we describe an illness primarily in terms of the nouns associated with it, we commit ourselves linguistically to making a diagnosis, the ultimate noun that fully captures the experience and hopefully unlocks the cure. This is a pretty fundamental part of our job, and if we run out of suitable diagnoses, we are free as a profession to develop new ones as needed. Constructs like Functional Neurological Disorder, Fibromyalgia, and Post-Traumatic Stress Disorder, however, only work if we can provide a convincing explanation of what is actually going on under the bonnet, and for this we need verbs. The benefit of using verbs to describe rather than nouns to define an illness is that it works even without a diagnosis, encourages ownership and naturally invites action. Of course, any consultation already involves the full spectrum of language, spoken and unspoken, and all of us have more than enough to be thinking about without analysing our sentence construction. If, however, you find yourself in a corner with a patient, and the focus is on things like *the pain, the leg, the diagnosis*, it might just be worth considering whether another way of speaking about the situation, expressed through actions, might help it to move on more smoothly.

Timber, Trees, and Sawdust[*]

Reality is continuous, but our experience of it is not. The earth turns smoothly, while our lives are split into day and night, work and play, sickness and health. Life is measured out according to familiar patterns and broken up by significant events like illness and pandemics, although it is often hard to see clearly where one part ends and the next begins. Did COVID-19 start when a novel coronavirus was identified in China in December 2019, or with the unknown first case before then; when the World Health Organization declared a pandemic on 11th March 2020, or when the British government announced a lockdown twelve days later? Did it finish when the last public restrictions in the UK were lifted two years after that, or when the WHO declared the situation no longer to be a public health emergency of international concern in 2023? Even now, people are still catching the virus, sometimes fatally, while others remain bereaved or affected by the ongoing consequences of earlier infection: the line between crisis and normality, event and continuum, is drawn at the level of our perception and behaviour as much as anything more concrete.[1]

Where we draw our lines makes a difference. Consider how anything potentially significant is distributed, whether it's disease cases around mobile phone masts, rocket damage to London during World War II, or common symptoms in the general population. If we look for them, it's impossible not to see cancer hot-spots, suspiciously intact neighbourhoods sheltering spies, and patients with any number of serious conditions. All are likely to be clustering illusions, arising through our tendency to collect

* An earlier version of this piece was published as: Hoban B. Seeing the timber and the trees. *Br J Gen Pract*. 2024 Oct 31;74(748):509. doi: 10.3399/bjgp24X739809. PMID: 39481893; PMCID: PMC11526747.

DOI: 10.1201/9781003652045-8

samples selectively, to divide up reality on the basis of what interests us rather than just letting it be.[2]

The problem, of course, is that if we are to grasp reality at all, we cannot let it be, but must categorise and name it in order to organise and make sense of our experience. We cannot survive without distinguishing between what is food and not food, safety and danger; or thrive without making a thousand other more subtle distinctions. It is therefore necessary on a daily basis that we cut across the grain of the world rather than simply running our hands along it, and yet with every stroke of the saw, we lose not just a little sawdust, but a little of our capacity to think in terms of the whole as well as its parts. We start with a tree and end up with timber.

Reductionism is a core feature of the scientific method, which, in the case of medicine, involves breaking down people into organs, organs into cells, and cells into molecules in order to understand them better. It has also come to involve isolating an individual from the dramatic arc of their life, stripping their story of context and disallowing any kind of meaning other than a strictly medical one: this is normal, that's abnormal; next patient please. The line between sickness and health is often indistinct, however, and in order to see it more clearly, it is essential that we look at the whole as well as the parts of someone's experience. The word *health* originally connotes wholeness, but its pursuit has come more and more to result in fragmentation; the fact that we can recognise integration as a function of general practice concedes the tendency of orthodox medicine to dis-integrate people.[3]

A purely reductionist approach is inherently dehumanising, addressing the substrate of someone's life rather than the life itself; unless doctor and patient also meet as fellow human beings, the results may be disappointing. And yet, whole-person medicine and continuity of care are not important because they add value to a strictly biomedical approach, but because patients are already whole people with continuous lives. Any approach that fails to recognise this necessarily falls short, offering at best an approximation of good care, and at worst a travesty of it. Rather than asking ourselves how much continuity we need in medicine, we should be considering how much discontinuity we can tolerate.

There is a tension, then, between viewing someone as a whole person, an individual capable of telling their own story, and as a collection of generic parts, whose malfunctions are best interpreted by experts. If we want to practise a mature, balanced sort of medicine, rather than one that sorts life into simple categories and only takes note of what can be counted and measured, we will never fully resolve this tension. We would do well, however, to look around us at the context in which we meet our patients, to note the continuity between one part of their life and another, and between ourselves and them, and sometimes to prefer listening and understanding to doing. A little sawdust here and there is inevitable, but too much, and one day there will be no more trees.

References

1. Robertson D, Doshi P. The End of the Pandemic Will Not Be Televised. *BMJ* 2021;375:e068094.

2. Howard Jonathan, *Cognitive Errors and Diagnostic Mistakes: A Case-based Guide to Critical Thinking in Medicine*. Springer, Cham, 2019.

3. Pereira Gray D. General Practice – The Integrating Discipline. *Br J Gen Pract* 2023. https://doi.org/10.3399/bjgp23X734697

Codes

How do you write up your consultations? Are you a template jockey, a fan of mysterious abbreviations and pithy one-liners, or does your typing speed allow you to expatiate in prose? *Little Jimmy entered the consulting room reluctantly, clutching his teddy while wiping away a dirty tear...*I'm regularly surprised on reading other doctors' entries in the notes how distinctive an individual's style can be, even when the subject matter is humdrum. For those who aspire to greater standardisation, this is, of course, anathema: the same problem should be described in the same way by any number of doctors, surely! The use of clinical codes encourages uniformity, and my software system even corrects my use of them – sorry, "offers preferred alternatives" – on a regular basis. When my medical imagination abandons me and all I can think to write after seeing a febrile child is *Viral illness*, the computer winks at me and logs instead *Viral disease*. I can hear Cecil Helman turn in his grave[1] and have to resist the urge to kick the PC, which is just as well, as it morphed from a large noisy box under my desk into a small quiet one on top of it a while ago: is this progress, or just a sign that machines are getting sneakier?

Clinical codes are, of course, created by the machines' human lackeys, but sometimes betray a way of thinking that is hard to relate to. *Nontraffic accident involving collision of motor-driven snow vehicle, not on public highway, rider of animal or occupant of animal-drawn vehicle injured (SNOMED-CT ID: 214704000)*, for example, is spot-on if you ever need to describe that event, but tells us little about the patient: are we talking about Lester Piggott or Father Christmas? It is as if someone had drunk too much coffee and tried to build a hyper-dimensional spreadsheet combining every possible medical and situational variable, and then fallen asleep halfway through.

DOI: 10.1201/9781003652045-9

Codes include diagnoses, disease constructs which are clearly defined and come as part of a standard package of symptoms, signs, investigations, differential diagnosis and treatment. From the perspective of general practice, there is something almost quaint about this: we spend so much of our time risk-managing non-specific presentations and wrestling with complexity that anything more straightforward feels like a throwback to simpler times, an oddity, or just an opportunity to claw back a few minutes in a late-running surgery. Medicine certainly seems more complicated now, a web of interconnected problems, and when we have to apply a label to something, it can be hard to know where to begin. I find myself using codes like *Frailty* and *Multiple symptoms* more often these days, a strategy that accommodates more under one roof and saves having to open a handful of tabs for each consultation.

There is perhaps in all of us a reasonable desire for accuracy and precision, but I think also an awareness that this approach has its limits. Sometimes precision comes at the expense of understanding, and it may be more useful to see a bigger picture at low resolution than a small one with crystal clarity. It is common for patients' notes to be littered with codes that reflect this: *Depression, Post-Traumatic Stress Disorder, Bereavement, Chronic alcoholism, Homelessness, Lost prescription*. Even these individual labels are just shorthand for a unique experience, but they huddle together on the summary screen, data points with a particular centre of gravity.

Ultimately, there may be many equally valid ways to code someone's problem, although it is worth considering that in deciding to use one code rather than another, we also commit ourselves to choosing one perspective over others. A diagnostic term (*Disorder of rotator cuff*) is conclusive but impersonal, while a descriptive one (*Shoulder pain*) is more tentative but focuses on what is most important to the patient. Headings referring to the cause of a presentation (*Motor vehicle traffic accident*) or its consequence (*Disability*) give a different point of view again. Of course, knowing who someone is and knowing them well are different things, and even the most meaningful code can only ever give us a limited amount of information. To a doctor who is familiar with their patient's story, however, the one code that takes into account all of it may simply be their name.

Reference

1. Helman C. Disease versus Illness in General Practice. *J R Coll Gen Pract* 1981;31:548–552.

Beware of Little Worlds

Generally speaking, we take what we see at face value, and, most of the time, we are right. Context is important, of course: we can enjoy watching an action film from the safety of our living room sofa precisely because we know it is not real. At other times, the context may be less clear, making it difficult to know how to react to the stranger trying to attract our attention or the raised voices in the next room. What is evident, though, is that our grasp of reality depends heavily on how we interpret the stream of incoming data from our senses, and that our brains are not merely passive receivers of the world's signal, but active generators of what we take to be the world. There is undoubtedly a reality outside our heads, but the one we deal with is inside them, a model that simulates it, shaping our expectations of what is outside and our responses to it. This model is not a smooth, shiny whole, but a diverse collection of experiences, assumptions and received wisdom held together with paperclips and string. Our perception of reality is necessarily flawed. Cognitive illusions and biases are not glitches in an otherwise perfect system, but the evidence of just how hard our brains work to make sense of the world around us.

It is inevitable, then, that our approximation of what is real and how things work sometimes lets us down, as when European visitors to Australia first came across black swans. There is a difference between the model and the reality, the map and the territory, and acknowledging this incongruence can be uncomfortable for us, like hearing a dissonant chord or looking at an Escher staircase that refuses to go properly up or down.[1] We like things to fit, to make sense, and we actively seek out congruence, like heliotropes following the sun or a cat stealing the comfy chair.

DOI: 10.1201/9781003652045-10

We do this partly by shrinking the world, sticking to situations with which we are familiar, and which we can therefore simulate more accurately. We also look for activities with clearly defined sets of goals, rules, rewards and penalties. Each of these represents a microcosm, a pocket universe in which things make sense, and in which success is clearly sign-posted and achievable. If you want to decide whether today was a good day, it's easy: Rashford scored; the profiteroles are perfect; you got past the boss fight. Any aspect of life can be stripped back to a simpler proposition in which we can immerse ourselves fully in order to experience congruence.[2]

We come across this stripping back in medicine. Addiction represents not just a chemical dependence or a pattern of behaviour, but also a smaller world in which priorities, needs and decision-making all come ready-made as part of the package, a template for life which makes more sense than the available alternatives, regardless of the consequences.[3] Some US Vietnam veterans, whose reality had come to be defined by trauma, experienced civilian life as constantly dissonant, and could only find a sense of wholeness, or congruence, by returning again and again to that trauma.[4] Autism seems to make it harder to model reality in general, rendering much of life incongruous and jarring.[5] If you can't make a map with which to navigate life, fixed routines and structure offer instead a safe and familiar path to guide the weary traveller home.

Medicine is itself a microcosm, a construct for making sense of the *disease* from which we all suffer at one point or another. There will always be discrepancies between how we feel and what we expect or understand, and sometimes these will be caused by one of the pathologies lined up in jars on the shelf at medical school. More often, they will simply reflect the limits of our perception: *we see through a glass, darkly*.[6] And yet, the sense of congruence we gain from thinking of what we feel as a *symptom* is so compelling that it can be difficult to know where to draw the borders of this little world.

We cannot manage without models, but it is easy to forget that they are not the same as reality, and that their utility depends not just on their ability to provide a sense of congruence, but on the degree to which they help us to engage meaningfully with the world around us. A good model is always a work in progress, which we refine by recognising its limitations. It is easy to become lost in our little worlds, and many of our patients have become lost in Medicine, which promises answers but often disappoints. If we are to be faithful guides in this world, we should take care to note its exits as well as its entrances.

References

1. Heath I. How Medicine Has Exploited Rationality at the Expense of Humanity. *BMJ* 2016;355:i5705. https://doi.org/10.1136/bmj.i5705 (Published 1 November 2016).

2. Csikszentmihalyi Mihaly, *Flow: The Psychology of Happiness*. Rider, London, 2002.

3. Dunnington Kent, *Addiction and Virtue: Beyond the Models of Disease and Choice*. Intervarsity Press USA, 2011.

4. van der Kolk Bessel, *The Body Keeps the Score: Mind, Brain and Body in the Transformation of Trauma*. Penguin, New York, 2015.

5. Barrett Lisa Feldman *How Emotions are Made: The Secret Life of the Brain*. Pan, New York, 2018.

6. The Bible, 1 Corinthians 13: 12, King James Version.

Avoiding Death

The BBC recently reported on "30,000 excess cardiac deaths in England" since the start of the COVID-19 pandemic, calculated as the difference between reported and expected deaths based on the previous five-year average.[1] This feels familiar from the regular televised briefings we had when coronavirus cast a longer shadow, although for a straightforward bit of arithmetic it covers a lot of ground. To start with, any statistical model is based on the assumption that what has happened so far is a guide to what will happen next, like deciding whether you'll need a jumper tomorrow because it was cold today. All things being equal, it may be a reasonable way to proceed, but we need to have some way of gauging whether they really are. If it's cold today and a tornado upends your house tomorrow, deciding what to wear will be the least of your worries. In the face of a global event like the COVID-19 pandemic, should we expect to be able to predict how many people die in a given week of a particular cause, and, when our prediction is different from what we measure, should we require the facts to justify themselves, as if they owed us an explanation for being unexpected, or should we check our assumptions?

The idea of excess deaths is, of course, just an attempt to make sense of what's happening in a complex system with a view to allocating resources appropriately. More interestingly though, the Office of National Statistics also publishes data relating to what are considered *avoidable* deaths, that is, those that *ideally should not occur in the presence of timely and effective healthcare*.[2] This rather loaded term includes deaths that could be avoided through public health or primary preventive measures, as well as those due to treatable conditions. It is anticipated that as healthcare becomes increasingly effective, more and more conditions will become either preventable or

DOI: 10.1201/9781003652045-11

treatable, and more deaths therefore avoidable; the most up-to-date figure for Great Britain currently stands at 22.8% of all deaths for 2020.[3] The intention is to use this metric to compare the effectiveness of different healthcare systems, which sounds like a good thing, although anyone who's ever been beaten over the head with performance-related statistics may already find themselves flinching.

Isn't this just a little bit weird? Unlike taxes, pretty much any death due to an identifiable cause can be considered avoidable in theory, whether it's caused by a car crash, avoidable through lower speed limits and safer car design, or a heart attack, through universal statin prescribing. Is it reasonable, though, to expect death to be the exception rather than the rule in life, as if we could insist that the Grim Reaper submit a business case to the authorities for approval before making his rounds? Even if we could, we are assuming that the job would fall to healthcare professionals, car manufacturers, or traffic legislators, when this seems largely not to be the case.

Most of the variation we see in health and longevity is due to factors not directly related to healthcare at all. We encourage our patients to eat well, keep active and not drink too much or smoke, but even this is mostly wide of the mark. If we looked at what primarily drives differences in health, we might say more honestly: don't be poor, disabled, or parent your child alone, and don't live in sub-standard accommodation or work in a stressful, low-paid manual job, but do make sure you get all the benefits you're entitled to and use your education to improve your socio-economic position.[4] Most people don't need more medicine to improve their health or live longer – they need a better life.

My final objection to classing deaths as avoidable is that it inevitably raises the question of culpability whenever someone dies. Webster's Duchess of Malfi declared that "...death hath ten thousand several doors for men to take their exits," but we risk cutting this down to just two, marked Failure and Old Age.[5] Is this really where we want to end up? There is naturally a place for well-informed professional reflection when any patient dies, or formal inquiry when an unusual pattern of deaths emerges, but it is surely in everybody's interest to go about this positively and with an open mind instead of trying to enforce statistically determined norms or necessarily attribute blame. The overall mortality rate will never fall below 100%, and however cunningly we avoid it, death is only ever postponed. It is unfortunate that ONS does not publish statistics on lives lived well, but maybe these are harder to come by.

References

1. NHS disruption driving rise in heart deaths, charity says, 3 November 2022, https://bbc.co.uk/news/health-63486547

2. Avoidable mortality in the UK QMI – Office for National Statistics, last revised 7 March 2022 https://ons.gov.uk/peoplepopulationandcommunity/healthandsocial care/causesofdeath/methodologies/avoidablemortalityinenglandandwalesqmi

3. Avoidable mortality in Great Britain: 2020 – Office for National Statistics. https:// ons.gov.uk/peoplepopulationandcommunity/healthandsocialcare/causesofdeath/ bulletins/avoidablemortalityinenglandandwales/2020

4. Marmot Michael, *The Health Gap: The challenge of an unequal world*. Bloomsbury, London, 2015.

5. Webster John, *The Duchess of Malfi*, Act 4, Scene 2, 1623.

How to Make a Decision

It's hard to go far online without being promised *The 7 Keys to Happiness, 10 Ways to Make People Like You,* or *3 Tips That Will Revolutionise Your Practice.* It seems unlikely that success in any of these areas can be reduced to a few transformative bullet points, and yet, it's hard to resist the allure of the headlines, with their subtext that the universe obeys a hidden code, and that if we only pay attention and do it right, everything will work out well for us.

The more obvious truth is that life is messy, uncertain, and full of ambiguities which must be negotiated with care. Deciding what to do is rarely clear-cut but depends instead on weighing up the likely costs, benefits and burdens of any course of action across multiple domains. This weighing-up is itself based on limited information viewed in the half-light of our own experience, priorities and available resources. This is the bigger picture in which we live, but we cannot constantly keep it in view without feeling overwhelmed: a world so complex and unpredictable is just too strange and threatening. As T.S. Eliot put it, *Human kind cannot bear very much reality.*[1] We all have to find a way of coming to terms with this, of dialling down reality so that day-to-day life becomes manageable, and bridging the gap between the things we know for sure and the decisions we need to make. Most decisions are not perfect, but they really only need to be good enough. If you want to make an accurate weather forecast, you're going to need a model and a lot of data and computing power, but if you just need to know what to wear to the shop, look out of the window.

Consider the consultation: a doctor may choose to follow their gut or rely on their knowledge of current guidance and best practice; they may prefer the consistency of always doing things the same way or the security of deferring to an expert; or they may simply do what is quickest, requires least effort or pleases their patient. All these approaches represent different

DOI: 10.1201/9781003652045-12

approximations, grids through which we strain our experience to catch the parts we can work with; *reality-lite*. Each of us looks at the same universe, but we see our own private worlds.

Patients are the same, giving us information which is necessarily incomplete, but intended to help us form a particular impression: *everything is okay really*; *something must be done*; *I'm falling apart*. Just as the same story can be told and understood in different ways, so the same patient might receive from one doctor reassurance, from another a prescription, and from a third, hospital admission. That may seem worryingly subjective, but it's certainly in keeping with experience.

How we decide to go about things depends largely on which brand of reality-lite we use. We can say as an article of faith that there is an objective world of appendicitis, asthma and brain tumours out there, while also recognising that our grasp of that world is less secure than we like to think, and that in practice things are often different to how they first seem. The key, perhaps, is not to be too attached to our own perspective, but to acknowledge it as one of many that may be more or less useful in a given scenario, and that may or may not match that of our patient.

The approximation we are taught at medical school is that patients are telling us their diagnosis.[2] Although this is true to a point, patients are generally saying more about their perspective than their pathology, in the same way that a ray of sunlight in a dark tool-shed tells us a little about how dusty the shed is, but much more about the sun.[3] The prerequisite to any successful communication is a basic agreement about what is being communicated, and it is easy to make assumptions about this that end up leading us astray. We may not inhabit the same experiential world as our patients, but we should at least be able to visit.

My killer tip to revolutionise your practice, then, is that the best way to make a decision is to do it together with the patient, not because they are right, or for the sake of being patient-centred, but because the origin and consequences of their problem play out in their world, and we are there as guests.

References

1. Eliot TS, Norton, Burnt, *Four Quartets*, 1944, first published by Faber & Faber Ltd.

2. Aronson JK, When I Use a Word…Listening to the Patient, *BMJ* 2022;376:o646.

3. Lewis CS. *Meditation in a Toolshed, Published in God in the Dock: Essays on Theology and Ethics*. Eerdmans, Grand Rapids, MI, 1970.

Narrative and Numbers*

Patients adopt a variety of approaches when talking to their doctor: they may tell a story, with all the contextual details that by turns help, hinder and misdirect; they may describe their symptoms, inviting us to provide an interpretation; they may name the problem, trusting that terms like *vertigo* and *wheeze* mean the same to both of us; or they may just quote numbers, that ultimate form of abstraction, whether referring to their blood pressure, their waistline, or how much pain they're in. Communication takes place across the whole of this spectrum, at one end rich in meaning but strictly personal, and at the other, precise but generic. As we move from narrative to numbers, we limit the opportunities for misunderstanding, but also for genuine understanding; we communicate more clearly, but we also communicate less.

This tension crops up in other areas too. The Quality and Outcomes Framework (QOF) considers only quantitative measures of patient care, for example. All things being equal, it is preferable to have lower rather than higher blood pressure, but not meeting a target could indicate either a poorly performing practice that doesn't know the rules, or an excellent one that looks beyond them and empowers patients to make their own decisions: there is complexity here which QOF points cannot adequately capture. Similarly, it is good to learn from our patients and colleagues, but the questionnaires approved for collecting feedback invite bland, standardised responses which generate another number: what does a percentage score really mean, other than that a test has been passed or failed? Does this really inform our learning? Patients attending an NHS health check are in

* An earlier version of this piece was published as: Hoban B. Narrative and numbers. *Br J Gen Pract*. 2024 Dec 26;75(750):33. doi: 10.3399/bjgp25X740469. PMID: 39725531; PMCID: PMC11684437.

DOI: 10.1201/9781003652045-13

the same position, having reached a point in life where age or changing circumstances prompt them to consider their health more carefully, and wanting to know where they stand. The outcome of their appointment, an estimate of 10-year cardiovascular risk, is so abstract that it can take considerable time to unpack, and the officially endorsed advice they receive reflects the wholesale price of statins more than any meaningful idea of whether they are in reasonable health for their age. Given the limited utility of numbers in healthcare, how is it that they have come to dominate our working life so much?

The most obvious answer is that we privilege a scientific, biomedical outlook, which views measurable realities as more valid than unmeasurable ones. Evidence-Based Medicine relies on quantifying the effectiveness of potential treatments in order to know which we should use. This is, of course, good in principle, but still depends on measuring meaningful outcomes in a representative group of patients: it doesn't necessarily tell us whether the person in front of us will benefit at all, or on whose terms. It is easy to find fault with what feel like more subjective approaches, but counting and measuring are prone to their own biases; the idea that basing decisions on numbers alone is somehow objective is in fact known as the McNamara fallacy.[1]

A natural consequence of this belief in the superiority of numbers is our tendency to measure things, even when it is unlikely to help. The *streetlight effect* calls to mind a home-owner who has lost their keys somewhere dark, but looks for them where the light is better.[2] When we look for a diagnosis by measuring someone's haemoglobin, liver function or whatever, and then reassure them that the results are normal, we are effectively saying that all is well, the keys can't be lost because we looked under the streetlight and couldn't find them! Faced with the needs of someone who is unaccountably fatigued, or in pain, or otherwise struggling with life, it is hard to gaze with them into the abyss and acknowledge our own helplessness; far easier to do some blood tests instead. The abstraction of numbers confers a certain distance from these everyday horrors, and a sense of agency in a job that often robs us of agency. Atul Gawande advised doctors who want to stay healthy and effective: *count something*.[3]

We walk a tightrope in medicine, balancing every day the unique and complex needs of individual patients with the standardised requirements of the rulebook that governs their care. There is danger in tipping too far in either direction, in concentrating too much on either the narrative or the numbers, but I believe that we are currently tipping towards the latter, and that this represents one element of the current crisis in the health service. The increasing use of laboratory investigations in primary care,[4] for example, generates significant additional work for everyone involved, but reflects a wider cultural shift from a more personal and nuanced model of care to one that is more scientific and intolerant of ambiguity. If we want to regain some measure of control over our working lives, we can either embrace this shift or push back against it. Knowledge, certainty and structure can all contribute to a sense of agency, but it is a contingent, brittle kind, which does not long survive contact with everyday life. A more robust variety grows instead from understanding, engagement and responsiveness to the needs of the people we are trying to help, and sometimes the numbers can be left to look after themselves.

References

1. Basler MH. Utility of the McNamara fallacy. *BMJ* 2009;339:b3141 https://doi.org/10.1136/bmj.b3141

2. Croskerry P. The Importance of Cognitive Errors in Diagnosis and Strategies to Minimize them. *Acad Med* 2003;78:775–780.

3. Gawande Atul, *Better: A Surgeon's Notes on Performance*. Metropolitan Books, New York, 2007.

4. Sullivan JW, Stevens S, Hobbs FDR, Salisbury C, Little P, Goldacre B et al. Temporal Trends in Use of Tests in UK Primary Care, 2000-15: retrospective Analysis of 250 Million Tests *BMJ* 2018;363:k4666. https://doi.org/10.1136/bmj.k4666

Illusions of Control

It is hopefully uncontroversial to say that doctors want to help, to improve the health of their patients. One of the great frustrations of the job, in fact, is the realisation that this isn't always possible, for the simple reason that those patients often have their own goals, or at least seem less committed to ours than we expected: they don't take their tablets, miss appointments, and refuse to follow the perfectly reasonable advice that we've given them. As with many things in life, healthcare would be easier if it didn't depend so much on other people, or if we could at least control their behaviour. If that makes you half-smile, it's because it's half-true; the other half is worth looking at more closely.

The urge to control is intrinsic to us as mammals: we are constantly engaged in homeostasis, adjusting our internal and external environments to maintain a thousand physiological parameters within narrow ranges. We register the difference between how things ought to be and how they are, and do what is necessary to close the gap: we put on a jumper, look for food, or give our adrenal glands a squeeze. We are often unaware of this process, but sometimes notice the incongruence that drives it, a perceptual itch that we try to scratch but cannot always reach. It is the same itch which leads us to nag our patients about their habits and their medication, although we are perhaps better at controlling our physiology than other people. The causal link between our actions and any outcome may be dubious, but the relief we feel at having done something, especially when there is an improvement of some kind, is so strongly reinforcing that we tend to ignore this. Our cognitive-behavioural homeostasis therefore readily gives rise to illusions of control: what I did must have worked because things seem better now.

DOI: 10.1201/9781003652045-14

Strictly speaking, illusions of control refer only to this imagined or inflated sense of our ability to influence outcomes.[1] We are prone to other illusions too, though, including the idea that control is possible in the first place. On a basic level, we can of course decide which shoes to put on in the morning, what class of antihypertensive to prescribe, or how to manage demand for appointments after a long weekend. Once we look beyond the immediate effects of these decisions, however, we may find that they have other consequences too: the shoes look good, but are uncomfortable and unconducive to home visits on foot; the tablets are out of stock, necessitating further communication and decision-making; prioritising the immediate availability of appointments can paradoxically worsen access in the longer term.[2] While it is therefore possible to alter outcomes in principle, simple interventions rarely have a predictable effect. If it is true that the purpose of a system is whatever it does, we should consider that the current performance of the NHS is fully in keeping with its design, even if this wasn't anyone's intention.[3]

The idea that medicine as a project is universally benign is illusory in the same way: there are certainly many outcomes that we can influence, but they are sometimes at odds with what matters most to patients. Where medicine was once the friend of the sick, it has now become the enemy of disease, and the doctor has changed from "an artisan exercising a skill on personally known individuals into a technician applying scientific rules to classes of patients."[4] Even the substrate of medicine is no longer the same: risk and metrics rather than symptoms, and subtle patterns only discernible by computers interrogating massive datasets. We have become part of a vast and restless mechanism whose purpose is to scratch the itch that we all feel, to exert control, and as with any itch, the more we scratch it, the more it bothers us.[5]

The acknowledged tension in general practice between treatment and prevention demonstrates that these represent not just two aspects of the same thing, but entirely different ways of dealing with people.[6] Medicine at its most basic is about caring for individuals in a way that helps them get on with their lives, but we risk making it instead a way of "managing proactively" those same individuals, controlling their blood pressure or cholesterol level, less for their own benefit than for the sake of so-and-so-many strokes prevented *per annum* or life years added to the faceless aggregate of humanity. Roy Campbell wrote: "I hate 'Humanity' and all such abstracts: but I love *people*," and it is difficult not to sympathise.[7]

The final illusion is that only those outcomes that we can in theory control are worthwhile, and that we help most by trying to achieve them on our patients' behalf. There is no question that modern medicine is immensely powerful, and yet it is too easy to become seduced by its power, to hide behind its smooth and certain walls and concern ourselves not with making sense of someone's individual needs, but with redefining those needs according to the help it is convenient for us to offer. If health is not just an abstract commodity, but the capacity to respond adaptively to illness in pursuit of something more meaningful, then we can never care for people simply by plugging them into the medical matrix.[8]

We should always want to help, and medicine equips us generously to do this. Ultimately, though, there is a limit to how much control we can exert over anyone's health, and there is a danger that by trying too hard to go beyond this, we foster instead a sense of fear, dependence and resentment in those we are trying to help. Life is, by its nature, uncertain, and we may do better to instil in our patients a degree of confidence and agency as they negotiate this than to offer them the illusion of certainty or control.

References

1. Thompson Suzanne C. Illusions of Control. In: Rüdiger F Pohl ed. *Cognitive Illusions: Intriguing phenomena in thinking, judgement and memory*. Routledge, Abingdon, 2017.

2. Voorhees J, Bailey S, Waterman H, Checkland K. A Paradox of Problems in Accessing General Practice: A Qualitative Participatory Case Study. *Br J Gen Pract* 2024;74(739):e104–e112. https://doi.org/10.3399/BJGP.2023.0276

3. "The purpose of a system is what it does," sometimes abbreviated to POSIWID, aphorism attributed to Stafford Beer (1926–2002).

4. Evans R. Ivan Illich's *Medical Nemesis* at 50. *Br J Gen Pract* 2025;75(750):26–27. https://doi.org/10.3399/bjgp25X740313

5. Sen A. Health: Perception Versus Observation. *BMJ* 2002;324:860–861.

6. Martin SA, Johansson M, Heath I, Lehman R, Korownyk C. Sacrificing Patient Care for Prevention: Distortion of the Role of General Practice. *BMJ*. 2025 Jan;21(388):e080811. https://doi.org/10.1136/bmj-2024-080811. PMID: 39837625.

7. Campbell Roy, *Light on a Dark Horse: An Autobiography*. Penguin, London, 1971.

8. Generalism Medical. *Now! Reclaiming the Knowledge Work of Modern Practice*, Joanne Reeve. CRC Press, Boca Raton, FL, 2023.

Swiss Cheese and the Power of Saying Sorry

When things go wrong in medicine, we are expected to learn and adapt our practice in order to protect patients.[1] Learning and adaptation are not unique to doctors, but it is perhaps worth considering what form they take in general practice in the wake of any kind of adverse event. Such events vary enormously, from the trivial or near-miss to something much more serious, and can generate strong feelings. Our response tends to follow a standard format, focussed on reestablishing the smooth running of the practice machinery: mistakes were made; lessons should be learnt; something must be done. Reasonable though this is in principle, it sometimes fails to address the real issues or the needs of those affected.

To start with, the complexity of healthcare means that it is generally easier to take token remedial action or attribute blame than to understand what has actually gone wrong. Even when proximate causes such as prescribing errors can be addressed, there are likely to be other factors behind them such as time pressure or conflicting directives, which are beyond our reach.

The Swiss Cheese Model describes how adverse events occur through an accumulation of system failures, like holes lining up in a stack of Emmental slices.[2] Responsibility for an event seems to lie with whoever made the last mistake, when it really belongs to a system that allows such errors to align in the first place. The way to stop things going wrong is to make the holes smaller, but what often happens instead is that the slices are simply rearranged: we can avoid repeating the same mistake, but only at the cost of making others.

Another snag in the tidy process of learning and adapting relates to how we approach cognitive bias, a system problem at the level of the human mind; individual, but also universal. Every diagnosis or decision we make

DOI: 10.1201/9781003652045-15

is arrived at cognitively, and each misdiagnosis or mistake is necessarily the endpoint of a cognitive process. It is tempting, therefore, to view these things as aberrations, when the reality is that thinking is an inherently risky business. The issue is not how to fix our mind so that it works properly, but how it works in the first place.

Consider the existence of pairs of complementary biases in our thinking, pulling us in opposite directions along the same axis. For example, *base rate neglect* means focussing on how well a diagnosis fits the case, regardless of how common or rare it is, while *Sutton's slip* involves choosing only the most obvious or prevalent diagnoses.[3] In fact, either "bias" acts as a counterweight to the other, ensuring that we take into account both the prevalence and the clinical features of a condition. Other examples broadly reflect tensions between the context and the content of a clinical encounter; we might do better to think of them simply as paired cognitive tendencies rather than biases. The lesson here is that our brain works as it does, and that error comes not from faulty thinking, but from a lack of balance or integration. In order to think clearly, we need to train our cognitive muscles, not restrain them.[4]

The idea that we can learn from our mistakes until we eventually stop making them is beguiling and clearly contains some truth. It also obscures a larger truth, however: just as holes and cognitive bias are intrinsic features of Swiss cheese and thinking, so there is a core of irreducible uncertainty in medicine; it is only ever in hindsight that we can claim to have all the answers.[5]

My final objection to viewing adverse events primarily in terms of learning is that we risk fundamentally mistaking the nature of healthcare: it is only incidentally a technical business; it is first of all interpersonal. By all means let us reflect and do better, but let us also recognise that when the wheels come off, we should still put people before process. We regularly emphasize the importance of relational care in general practice, and it is perhaps inevitable that when things go wrong, the resulting pain is felt, and expressed, at a relational level. The danger of trying to avoid this is that the learning process becomes a means either for doctors who feel guilty to hide from their patients, or for patients who feel let down to punish their doctors. GPs, many of whom already suffer from Impostor Syndrome, may see themselves as helpless in this situation, victims of circumstance, as indeed may their patients.[6] There is power, though, in an apology made in good faith, and power in accepting one; both demonstrate that we can still work together in the light of our shared and fallible humanity. It is obviously best to avoid making the same mistake twice, but we cannot honestly promise not to make others in future. Our response to an adverse event may include learning and change, but it should always recognise too the things we cannot change, promote a better understanding of what happens between our ears, and affirm the relationships on which we depend to navigate a dysfunctional system in an uncertain world.

References

1. Openness and honesty when things go wrong: The professional duty of candour, GMC,http://gmc-uk.org/professional-standards/the-professional-standards/candour---openness-and-honesty-when-things-go-wrong/encouraging-a-learning-culture-by-reporting-errors

2. Reason J. The Contribution of Latent Human Failures to the Breakdown of Complex Systems. *Phil Trans R Soc Lond B* 1990;327475–327484. https://doi.org/10.1098/rstb.1990.0090

3. Crosskerry P. The Importance of Cognitive Errors in Diagnosis and Strategies to Minimize Them. *Acad Med* 2003;78:775–780.

4. Ryle, Cym Anthony, *Risk and Reasoning in Clinical Diagnosis: Process, Pitfall and Safeguards*. Oxford University Press, Oxford, 2019.

5. Han Paul KJ, *Uncertainty in Medicine: a Framework for Tolerance*, Oxford University Press, Oxford, 2021.

6. Bravata DM, Watts SA, Keefer AL, Madhusudhan DK, Taylor KT, Clark DM, Nelson RS, Cokley KO, Hagg HK. Prevalence, Predictors, and Treatment of Impostor Syndrome: A Systematic Review. *J Gen Intern Med.* 2020 Apr;35(4):1252–1275. https://doi.org/10.1007/s11606-019-05364-1. Epub 2019 Dec 17. PMID: 31848865; PMCID: PMC7174434.

The Cliff and the Bog

I'd like you to imagine that you're out walking in the countryside; probably you've taken some annual leave because it's quite a remote spot, the sort of place that takes time and planning to find. It's a fine day, and you're not rushing, but you know that you want to reach wherever it is that you're headed before it gets dark. You're following a track downhill when something catches your eye, perhaps a butterfly, and in the time it takes you to readjust your focus, you realise that the path has petered out and the scenery changed. On your left the grass now runs to a sheer drop, past which you can see only blue sky, although you can hear the boom and crash of waves against cliffs far below. On your right the ground is firm for a little way, but soon becomes waterlogged and boggy, ready to steal your boots and coat you in thick, chocolatey mud. You walk along easily enough for a while, noticing that the sun is already a little lower than it was, when out of nowhere a thick white mist rolls in, blocking out sight and sound around you. You wait for a moment, but nothing changes, and you realise that you're in a spot of bother. You need to keep going, but stray too far to the left and you'll be over the cliff edge before you know it; go too far to the right and you'll be bogged down, and who knows what state you'll be in if you ever reach your destination? Avoid one danger and you'll be risking the other. Just then, it strikes you that your situation is a picture of two contrasting dangers that doctors face every day of their professional lives: misdiagnosis and over-medicalisation.

The idea that medicine can heal all ills does not long survive contact with the reality of chronic pain, adverse circumstances, frailty and progressive disease. Most patients, and most doctors, accept this on the understanding that we should at least be able to recognise those conditions that

DOI: 10.1201/9781003652045-16

are either treatable or have the potential to alter the trajectory of their lives: cancer, sepsis, heart disease, neurodegenerative conditions and so on. Stories of missed diagnosis in which the doctor was too rushed, uninformed or closed-minded to recognise what they were dealing with are the constant background noise of medical practice, and nobody wants to be that doctor. We can all tell stories of patients who seemed well enough at the time but turned out later to have something terrible, and, especially when we've had our fingers burnt, we naturally practise with a degree of caution.

Our training as doctors equips us primarily to look for pathology in our patients, and the pressure not to miss a diagnosis inevitably heightens this, so that when faced with atypical or ambiguous presentations, we default to seeing disease. Even if we allow for this, it can be difficult to know how much uncertainty to tolerate; an honest answer to the question *Could this be cancer?* is rarely a straight No. As a result, the threshold for investigation has now fallen to a point where incidental findings like mildly abnormal liver function tests or lung nodules have become much more common than genuine abnormalities related to the reason our patient consulted us in the first place.[1, 2]

Putting these things to bed takes a significant amount of time, work and worry for doctors and patients, and it is reasonable to ask whether our current practice still represents a good balance of benefits, burdens and risks. More crucially, have we reached a point where the noise in the system makes it harder to recognise the signal, and where our frantic activity actually becomes a barrier to patient care? If I spend the whole consultation making sure that my patient doesn't have cancer, will I pick up her parkinsonian tremor or have time just to listen? And if doctors find it so difficult to pass patients as healthy, how can we expect patients ever to have enough confidence in their health to stop worrying and get on with life? We tend to think of clinical risk as applying to high-impact cases in which an individual clinician drops the ball and a patient comes to harm. The less visible and arguably far greater risk comes from a system that overloads itself by promoting nosological hyper-vigilance, while disempowering patients without doing anything to help them manage their experience of illness.

Let's return to our walk in the mist between the cliff and the bog, misdiagnosis and over-medicalisation. We should be clear by now that there is no risk-free option, only a choice between different risks, and that the only way to avoid one entirely is to move towards the other. How we navigate this landscape will vary based on our past experiences, circumstances and general outlook on life; it will also make a difference to our effectiveness as doctors, our satisfaction at work, and the amount of baggage we end up taking home with us. Indeed, the point of the walk is not exclusively to avoid danger, but to cover ground, to get on, and hopefully enjoy the exercise. I would like to suggest that the point of doctors is not just to diagnose disease, but also to protect patients from a system that risks making the diagnosis of disease its only concern, and to help them thrive amidst the daily uncertainties of life. Finding a space in which to walk with our patients that acknowledges the dangers on both sides should benefit us all.

References

1. O'Sullivan M. Grigg and Ioannidis, Prevalence and Outcomes of Incidental Imaging Findings: Umbrella Review. *BMJ* 2018;361:k2387. https://doi.org/10.1136/bmj.k2387

2. Cancer Research UK Early Cancer Diagnosis Data Hub crukcancerintelligence.shinyapps.io/EarlyDiagnosis/ (accessed 29 October 2022).

Imaginary Medical Solutions[*]

One of our suppliers recently introduced a series of innovative measures designed to improve their customer experience, as a result of which they now only deliver once a week, and I found myself double-parked at the wrong end of the high street, having to pick up a new defibrillator. We had decided to cancel our usual surgery Christmas dinner on planetary health grounds, in favour of a cold-water chanting retreat, but I'd managed to get out of it by pleading an imminent risk to service provision if we didn't replace the old defib. I'm sure it's fine, even if the generator handle does get a bit stiff charging to 360J, but the Care Quality Commission were very particular about it at their last visit. There was a notice on the supplier's door announcing that they were shut, apparently as part of an exciting programme of changes to their consumer-facing presence that would enhance something or other. So there I was, wondering what to do, when I noticed the shop next door. It had a flaking hand-painted sign announcing it as Imaginary Medical Solutions, and a window display that invited deep cleaning rather than curiosity. I don't remember going inside, but I must have done, because all of a sudden I was looking out through the window rather than in; the bell over the door hung silently, declining comment. As if by magic, the shopkeeper appeared. "Looking for anything in particular today, Sir, or just browsing?" He was a plump, comfortable-looking man in pin-striped trousers and a plain shirt, with a purple waistcoat and matching fez, and I had the feeling I'd seen him before somewhere. He must have noticed, because he smiled and said, "I know, I have one of those faces. Let me show you around."

[*] An earlier version of this piece was published as: Hoban B. Imaginary Medical Solutions. *Br J Gen Pract*. 2024 Nov 28;74(749):554. doi: 10.3399/bjgp24X740061. PMID: 39609064; PMCID: PMC11611333.

DOI: 10.1201/9781003652045-17

The shop didn't seem to have a layout, so much as a foreground, middle ground and background, with stacked wooden packing crates framing a collection of apparently random objects of various sizes displayed on every available surface. I picked up what looked like a Blackberry with three separate screens and keyboards, thinking that it seemed just a touch excessive. "It's a Universal Communicator, Sir, with dedicated inputs for text, context and subtext. Very popular, never get your wires crossed again!" Next to it was an odd-looking curved length of polished wood, with a cork handle at one end and a fountain-pen nib at the other. "That one is a Narrative Arc: you line it up with the elements of the story you have already and mark off where it's likely to end. Nowadays most people prefer to use a Retrospectoscope, although if you're interested in the past, you may also want to consider a Biographical Strain Gauge." He reached up to a precariously balanced shelf and brought down what looked like a jazzed-up Geiger counter, with a base unit connected by a flex to some kind of sensor. "It detects traces of loss, hardship and vulnerability; you'll have to turn up the sensitivity from the factory setting, though, or you won't pick up much."

The shopkeeper was clearly getting into his stride, and as it seemed unlikely that he'd have anything as mundane as resuscitation equipment, I decided to go with the flow. The glasses he produced seemed a bit more ordinary, although I wondered if they'd once had a fake nose and moustache attached. "Gestalt Spectrometer," he pronounced as he snapped the case shut. "Lets you see what sort of patient you're dealing with before you get into the details. I would leave that one alone though, Sir." Without thinking, I'd picked up what looked like a Möbius strip made out of magnetic tape. "It's a conversational loop, a byproduct of dysfunctional speech, totally pointless." "Really?" I replied, intrigued. "Yes, best avoided." "How come?" I asked him. "You just end up going round in circles. It's a conversational loop, you see, a byproduct of dysfunctional speech, pointless, best avoided…" The shopkeeper was frowning. I was about to ask him about the loop thingy when he took my arm rather forcefully and marched me off to the till.

"Sorry about that," he said, having regained his composure. "Allow me to throw in an Adjustable Frame of Reference to make up for any unpleasantness. The invoice will be in the post." On the counter was a sturdy-looking carrier bag filled with brown paper packages. I hadn't seen an assistant anywhere, but somebody must have been very efficient with the scissors and string while I was being shown around. I looked up from the counter to tell the shopkeeper I hadn't intended to buy anything, but only saw my own reflection in the display window as I stood on the pavement outside, with the bag at my feet. I could hear carol singers somewhere in the distance.

The surgery was cold and empty when I got back, and I sat in the office with a cup of tea, going through my apparently real medical solutions. As I unpacked the Adjustable Frame of Reference, I decided that getting roughed up by the shopkeeper hadn't been so bad really, and a freebie is a freebie after all. There was one last package in the bag that I didn't recognise. I undid the string and unwrapped a heavy, bright yellow plastic case, labelled: "Automated Empathic Defibrillator, attach electrodes to both parties and activate when instructed! Warning, transfer immediately to nearest Continuous Care Unit (CCU) once rapport has been re-established!"

Since then, our supplier has undergone a radical restructuring, leading to a dynamic redeployment of resources and the termination of its local service. Maybe another trip to Imaginary Medical Solutions is in order.

PART II

How the System Works

As doctors, we generally think of our role in terms of the consultation, although we recognise that this takes place within the local context of the practice, the wider context of the health service as a whole, and the global context of medical research, the manufacture and distribution of medicines, and the training and recruitment of healthcare professionals. Many patients express profound thanks that at a time of serious illness, when they fell unexpectedly over the edge of their everyday lives, they were caught and held, not by any one individual, but instead by the safety net represented by this extensive system, of whose existence they had always been aware, but on which they hadn't previously needed to rely.

A net, or network, is a useful picture of the health service, in which different individuals and groups of people appear as nodes connected to each other in specific ways, so that a patient entering the network at a given point can pass from one node to another until they reach the one appropriate to their situation. One of the key features of this network in our case is that it is deliberately built around general practice, which limits and directs the flow of patients from primary to secondary care so that the system functions smoothly and everyone gets what they need.

Just as general practice prioritises the patient's agenda, and is therefore by definition patient-led, or, from the point of view of the system, reactive, so the emphasis of secondary care is much more on excluding or treating disease, and hence intrinsically doctor-led, and proactive. This differentiation is healthy, but assumes a balance of numbers which favours GPs over consultants, so that the system as a whole is driven by the priorities of the

DOI: 10.1201/9781003652045-18

people using it. Although it is well recognised that there are too few GPs working in the NHS, the number of doctors overall is steadily increasing. The problem is therefore not simply that we are under-doctored, but that the balance between generalist and specialist care has changed, leading to a change in outlook. A number of trends within general practice have amplified this effect: an increase in remote consulting prompted by the COVID-19 pandemic; the promotion of non-medical practice through the Additional Roles Reimbursement Scheme; and the gradual rise in list sizes as smaller practices close or merge.

The outcome in practical terms is an increasingly fragmented system focussed on preventing, identifying and fixing pathology. Whatever the merits of this system, it is often a hostile environment for the kind of relational, patient-centred care traditionally associated with general practice. A safety net implies distance: it is enough for us to know that it is there, far below us, so that we can focus instead on the high wire or trapeze without having to worry about falling. As the network representing the health service changes, this distance is shrinking, and many of our patients are instead becoming tangled in the net. They are exposed to iatrogenic harm and losing confidence in their health, learning to become afraid of disease without being enabled to live well or pursue the things that matter most to them.

It is clear that our efforts to make the system more consistent, productive and efficient are already changing its character. We may not be able to predict where this will ultimately lead, but it is not difficult to imagine the kinds of dystopian future healthcare that we would all prefer to avoid. Perhaps the challenge is to understand better the branching pathways in the network of our decision-making, so that the changes we make in good faith today don't leave us in a worse position tomorrow.

The USP of General Practice

One of the biggest changes in UK general practice over the last twenty years has been the entry of other primary care professionals into what used to be exclusively a doctor-and-nurse shop. These new colleagues are now regularly involved with, and sometimes lead the management of, acute illness, long-term conditions, antenatal care, and musculoskeletal and mental health problems. They consult, examine, prescribe, visit, write fit notes, review medication, arrange radiological investigations and refer to secondary care, while receptionists help patients to navigate this new landscape and practice managers oversee it. Integrated IT systems mean that we are no longer the only ones with access to a patient's medical past, and clever software can spot patterns of disease and keep up to date on current guidance better than we can. The only thing we do uniquely as GPs is to issue death certificates, although the newly introduced Medical Examiners may decide at some point that this is more within their remit. If no element of our portfolio is ours alone, are we still needed, or are we on the path of the dinosaurs, great in their day but now preserved only in museums?

The lack of a proprietary function is perhaps debatable. Although one competent clinician can manage this or that disease as well as another, what of the patients whose difficulties defy diagnosis: are they destined to orbit forever the outpatient department of the local hospital, passing from one baffled consultant to another? And what of those with multiple problems, including social and emotional domains as well as the merely medical? Ought they to be looked after by an army of specialists or by one sympathetic generalist?

DOI: 10.1201/9781003652045-19

Medical training and practice are based on the biomedical model, which conceives of people fundamentally as wet machines, whose malfunction generates an error code of symptoms and signs that a suitably qualified practitioner can interpret with a view to fixing the problem. Experience and professional disappointment tell us that things are often a good deal more complicated than this model allows, and yet we still have an obligation to care for our patients: how then can we manage the gap that often exists between what we read in our textbooks and what we see in our surgeries? It is our privilege as GPs to deal with the person behind the illness, whether they have one diagnosis, a dozen, or none at all. Indeed, if we have a Unique Selling Point as doctors, it may simply be that we are able and willing to work outside the biomedical model when the situation demands it. It's not that we necessarily carry out any tasks that other clinicians cannot, but that our involvement in the lives of our patients, and our ability to help them, do not depend on making either a specific diagnosis, or indeed any diagnosis. Our role depends instead on being able to consider their perspective as well as our own. We have one foot in the medical world, and another in that of everyday life, enabling us to bridge the gap between them.

GPs are not good at relational care or managing complexity and uncertainty because of any inherent aptitude for these things, but because our role places us into an environment in which they are unavoidable. A paramedic or pharmacist could, in principle, do the same, but may less often have the opportunity, or indeed the expectation, of doing so. In some ways, then, the question is not so much whether we still need GPs, but whether we still want the kind of continuous generalist healthcare to which general practice has always aspired, regardless of who provides it. If we do, then opening the doors to other practitioners needn't signal the weakening of our brand or our imminent extinction. Instead, we can consider how to become more involved in the training and supervision of these professionals so that they are ready to work effectively alongside us. The danger otherwise is that as the number of GPs falls, the outlook and practice of those who remain will instead come to resemble those of their more biomedically-oriented colleagues, and we will lose the very thing that currently makes us distinctive.

Hummingbirds and Foxes*

GPs do very little nowadays that could be described as routine. Practice nurses, healthcare assistants, midwives and pharmacists have been looking after this side of patient care for a long time, and, more recently, mental health and wellbeing practitioners, first contact physiotherapists, nurse practitioners, paramedics and advanced care practitioners have been managing much of the more acute and non-routine care in general practice too. Given the shortage of doctors, this seems both reasonable and practical, and frees up GPs to deal with what's left. Let's be honest here: looking after patients nowadays is governed far more by guidelines of some kind or other than used to be the case, and our core strength probably hasn't ever been the ability to follow rules.

Where does this leave us, then? Can we still argue that it's right for us to manage everything from tonsillitis to terminal care personally in order to nurture the cherished doctor–patient relationship, or should we focus on those elements of care that are too complex or poorly defined to fit within the portfolio of our colleagues? Can we still reasonably describe ourselves as generalists, doing a bit of everything, or are we on the road to re-branding ourselves as specialists in primary care?

A hummingbird is a specialist, highly adapted to hover in front of a flower and extract nectar from it. It does this extremely effectively, and looks amazing doing it, but is limited to a very specific setting in which its adaptations will work. A fox, by contrast, is very much the generalist, at home in a variety of settings, and particularly able to exploit the opportunities which our

* An earlier version of this piece was published as: Hoban B. Hummingbirds and Foxes. *Br J Gen Pract.* 2023 Aug. 31;73(734):421. doi: 10.3399/bjgp23X734913. PMID: 37652735; PMCID: PMC10471342.

DOI: 10.1201/9781003652045-20

modern urban environment offers an omnivorous species. Foxes are liminal, scruffy chancers sneaking around among the dustbins under cover of dark.

GPs are liminal too, practising on the threshold between the medical and the everyday. We rarely dazzle with our clinical acumen. Rather, we help our patients to negotiate the gloomy landscape of ill health and make good decisions when there are no perfect ones, sharing with them the uncertainty of the world outside the guidelines. There is much well-intentioned guess-work, and experience is measured in lessons learned from our mistakes. By and large, patients are looking for someone they can trust to do their best, rather than a wizard with all the answers.

We will never be specialists in the sense of either the hummingbird or our colleagues in secondary care. Our strength lies not in being able to do one thing perfectly, but in doing many things effectively in the grey zones of medicine, where others cannot survive. Physicians deal in *physic* and surgeons work with their hands,[1] but the GP's role is a function of the inability of either branch of the profession to meet patients' needs in isolation. And yet, despite our obligate generalism, we still act as consultants in the sense that other professionals within the practice team consult and refer patients to us.

If a re-branding is in order, then, how about Consulting Primary Care Generalists? As the role of non-medical clinicians in our practices continues to grow, we are well-placed to lead, oversee and support these colleagues, whose scope of practice is more restricted and closely bounded by protocols: it may be that we are now needed less to see every patient and deal with every problem, and more to provide the generalist overview that gives general practice its cohesion. Such a reconfiguring of our role would certainly reduce direct patient contact and personal continuity of care, which have always been as much a part of what we do as generalism. When we talk of a crisis in general practice, it is therefore in the sense not just of a time of great difficulty, but of a moment of decision, when things could go either one way or the other. Even if we double medical school places tomorrow, can we really wait another decade for a new generation of doctors to enter practice?

The current realities may mean that rather than holding on for an increase in our numbers to maintain the status quo, we consider instead other ways of upholding the distinctive features of general practice, and how a smaller number of GPs might make the most effective use of their skills and experience alongside colleagues from a variety of professional backgrounds. In this context, it would make sense to lengthen rather than shorten medical and general practice training, while aligning the training of non-medical clinicians more closely with general practice. Resilience is not just about personal toughness, but also about adapting as a profession to changing circumstances, and foxes are survivors.

Note

1 *Physic* is an archaic term for medicine. *Surgeon* is derived from *chirurgeon*, which is itself derived from the Greek words *cheir*, meaning a hand, and *ergon*, meaning work: hence, someone who works with their hands.

One Big Thing[*]

Something that becomes apparent after working for a while in General Practice is that we do lots of different things, but also One Big Thing. You can make a list of the different things: managing acute illness, diagnosing serious diseases like cancer, helping people with long-term conditions including functional disorders and mental health problems, offering support to the frail and isolated, doing the odd practical procedure, supervising assorted learners and non-medical staff, filling out forms and providing informal advocacy, digging through the drifts of pathology results and correspondence that accumulate silently overnight, and attending meetings of dubious utility. The One Big Thing is harder to put a finger on, but sometimes suggests itself through the other things that cause us frustration when they get in its way, or in the feeling of weary satisfaction at the end of a busy day that sometimes still reminds us that we do a good job.

There is certainly a lot to do each day, and we are spread more thinly than before. The widespread recruitment of Additional Roles Reimbursement Scheme clinicians within Primary Care Networks assumes that there is a core of work which is best left to GPs, and a negotiable periphery that we can delegate to others. The line between the core and the periphery is then necessarily drawn at the point where standard protocol-driven care gives way to the individualised management of patients with more complex needs. If demand in the system were fixed, this division of labour would lead to a smaller number of GP appointments, which would be more challenging but potentially also more rewarding – and, of course, longer. Tea and biscuits

[*] An earlier version of this piece was published as: Hoban B. One Big Thing. *Br J Gen Pract*. 2024 Mar 27;74(741):172. doi: 10.3399/bjgp24X736881. PMID: 38538127; PMCID: PMC10962505.

DOI: 10.1201/9781003652045-21

would be lovely, thank you. Alas, demand appears to be unlimited, so the extra help risks leading instead to an increase in the complexity and intensity of our work, without creating any additional time in which to do it.[1]

The idea of core and peripheral GP workload has an intuitive appeal, but breaks down under scrutiny. Look closely at the different things we do, and there is very little that could not in theory be done by someone else. Our ability to manage complex problems is not some kind of superpower, for which our regular low-level involvement with patients is merely the cover, like the superhero's day job. Rather, this more routine work is the foundation of our relationships with patients, and lends context to higher-level care when it becomes necessary. We learn our craft not by studying complexity, but by getting to know people. We are not ultimately specialists in complex care, but generalists whose role emerges from a diversity of tasks, even though most are straightforward when viewed in isolation.[2]

Emergence refers to systems whose properties go beyond a simple scaling-up of the properties of their components, such that the behaviour of the whole is not readily predictable from a knowledge of the parts.[3] Just as neighbourhoods with their own character emerge from particular arrangements of buildings, people and services, our One Big Thing emerges from a workload that is necessarily varied. Take away any one element and the effect may not be significant, but keep taking away more, and at some point, the character of the whole will change. If what we do as GPs contains no essential core, then it can have no dispensable periphery either, and delegating work to others may just mean that we become less involved with our patients, and therefore less effective. Does this matter, or is occasional "quality time" spent dealing with people's weightier concerns enough to maintain good working relationships and a generalist outlook?

GPs have always worked alongside other professional and informal caregivers, and there has never been a time when we could meet all our patients' needs ourselves: there is therefore no reason in principle why we cannot share out some of our workload within practices and Primary Care Networks (PCNs). It is worth reflecting, however, that current trends may be leading us not towards some kind of magical core role, but merely away from our roots. Generalism is primarily about integration rather than complexity,[4] and if we want to maintain our professional character and avoid making our working days even more difficult, we need to consider carefully how to avoid fragmenting our role by delegating its parts, and how instead to support our new colleagues in adopting a more generalist approach themselves.

References

1. Khan N. The Complex Consultation – Are We Seeing More Complex Patients and Why? *BJGP Life* 2023. http://bjgplife.com/the-complex-consultation-are-we-seeing-more-complex-patients-and-why/

2. Reeve Joanne, *Medical Generalism, Now!* CRC Press, Boca Raton, FL, 2023.

3. Johnson Steven, *Emergence: The Connected Lives of Ants, Brains, Cities and Software*. Penguin, London, 2002.

4. Pereira Gray D. General Practice – The Integrating Discipline. *Br J Gen Pract* 2023. https://doi.org/10.3399/bjgp23X734697

Facing Both Ways

It's generally accepted that you can't stop progress, but also that they don't make 'em like they used to. We aspire simultaneously to the values of a brighter future and those of a rosier past, buying cheap mass-produced stuff online while happily paying a premium for artisanal goods at a weekly market. Which way we face depends on context: imagine taking someone to a fancy restaurant and finding a stack of ready meals on the side with instructions for re-heating, or needing to replace your phone and visiting a workshop for the components to be machined and assembled by hand to produce a unique device.

We see the same in medicine. Ever since the 1950 Collings report examined standards in British General Practice,[1] there has been a move towards care that is increasingly consistent, organised and evidence-based, regardless of whether it is provided by an individual doctor, any doctor, or a non-medical clinician. In contrast to this progressive view, we are now also looking back to a time when continuity of personal care could be assumed, and lamenting its loss in the light of all its acknowledged benefits.[2]

General Practice, then, shares the values of both the dinner date and the mobile phone, and this is reflected in the way patients consult differently depending on context, preferring ease of access for simple acute problems and continuity of care for complex ongoing ones.[3] Broadly speaking, this corresponds to situations in which we deal primarily with either the standardised biomedical model of *disease*, or the individual psycho-social experience of *illness*,[4] although there is considerable overlap.

The recognition that General Practice has included a lot of routine, uncomplicated and non-clinical tasks, while GPs are a limited, highly trained and relatively expensive workforce dealing with ever-rising demand,

DOI: 10.1201/9781003652045-22

has led to the delegation of much of our workload to others within the practice team and the wider NHS. This naturally raises the question of whether, as we look ahead to the future, people will still need GPs, or whether we'll all soon be replaced by machines.[5] Looking back, though, we can reflect that we are not machines ourselves, nor do we simply operate the machinery of healthcare; we are the ghosts in the machine that allow it to become more than the sum of its parts.

The majority of consultations in General Practice do not map well onto specific care pathways or evidence-based guidelines. Instead, we get our bearings and direction of travel from our patients' perspective, and the information on which we base our diagnosis and management comes mostly from listening and talking to them, a less robust or reproducible process than some might like. Even when a diagnosis is clear, we treat individuals, not populations, and guidelines are written for the mean rather than the majority.

As a result, we are left with a large residue of uncertainty which must somehow be carried, like a sofa or a piano, by both parties working together. The doctor holds their end by expending time, attention and care on the patient's behalf; the patient holds theirs by accepting an element of risk and retaining responsibility for their own health. This is partly why it can be difficult to manage undifferentiated presentations remotely. Seeing a patient face to face is usually more informative; crucially, however, it also demonstrates a greater expenditure of effort and goodwill on the doctor's part, prompting a reciprocal willingness on the patient's to accept that things may not be clear-cut or fixable. The management of uncertainty, like so much, is largely relational.

It costs a computer nothing to tell patients to keep an eye on things for a bit longer: they must simply decide whether or not to accept the advice on its merits and bear the consequences. A non-medical clinician can go the extra mile to engage their confidence, but only along the well-marked paths of evidence and protocol. GPs operate in the wilderness beyond, often at significant cost to their own wellbeing. We are artisans, but we learn our craft through years on the assembly line. It is inevitable that our role will continue to change, but by owning both sets of professional values we can ensure that we face the future – and the past – with confidence.

References

1. Collings LS. General Practice in England Today. A Reconnaissance. *Lancet* 1950;i:555–585.

2. Pereira-Grey D, Sidaway-Lee K, White E, et al. Improving Continuity: THE Clinical Challenge. *InnovAiT* 2016;9(10):635–645.

3. Baker R, Boulton M, Windridge K, Tarrant C, Bankart J, Freeman GK. Interpersonal Continuity of Care: A Cross-sectional Survey of Primary Care Patients' Preferences and Their Experiences, *BJGP* 2007;57:283–290.

4. Helman C. Disease versus Illness in General Practice. *Journal of the Royal College of General Practitioners*, 1981;31:548–552.

5. Armitage R. The Moravec Paradox and Its Application in Health Care. *BJGP Life* 29 July 2023.

Looking In and Looking Out[*]

How we define health is one of those old chestnuts which invite regular debate, even though – or indeed because – it's difficult to agree on an answer. The question that is related but less often asked is not *what*, but *where* health is. When we measure the level of haemoglobin in someone's blood, or outline their organs using the latest form of radiological magic, the answer seems clear: inside the body. To the elderly widower coming to terms with the loss of his life partner, it is just as clearly different: health is outside too, in the ties that bind us to each other, and whose severing leaves us not just alone, but diminished.

Throughout medical history, there has been a tension between systems that locate health within the patient and those that have it outside. We consider the orthodox western approach normative, while perhaps dabbling a bit in complementary therapies like acupuncture or chiropractic. All are similar, however, in viewing the body as the place where things go wrong, and where they must be put right, whether we think in terms of the circulation of oxygenated blood, the flow of energy or the correct alignment of the vertebrae. This view may seem so self-evidently correct to us that it's difficult to think of an alternative, but some traditional forms of medicine have tended to look outside the body at its wider context, seeing health as a state of harmony between the body and society, nature, and the supernatural world, however these are construed.[1] Viewed from this perspective, health is simply one aspect of a life lived well within the matrix of the universe rather than a property of bodies – or minds – in isolation.

[*] An earlier version of this piece was published as: Hoban B. Looking in and looking out. *Br J Gen Pract*. 2024 Feb 29;74(740):132. doi: 10.3399/bjgp24X736701. PMID: 39222441; PMCID: PMC10904110.

DOI: 10.1201/9781003652045-23

We see vestiges of this tension in the modern conflict between theories of nature and nurture in determining who we are, between the biomedical and psychosocial models of ill health, and between objective, measurable indicators of disease and subjective, constructed narratives of illness. At the heart of these differences is the same question: Can we understand someone better by peering inside, or by examining instead how they relate to the world around them?

As with most dichotomies, there is, of course, value on both sides. Our current healthcare system rates looking in much more highly than looking out, however, as demonstrated by the constant quest for greater diagnostic precision through the use of blood tests and scans.[2-4] Having to discuss with someone how they're feeling or what their concerns might be can seem a little outdated. Our implicit aspiration is for the technology to relate directly to the disease, bypassing the patient, the doctor, and any kind of relationship between them. While science clearly has its place in medicine, there is a danger that we are cultivating a kind of medical esotericism, in which truth becomes the preserve of an inner circle of wizard-priests, and knowledge is power. In this sense, professional medicine always runs the risk of disempowering those it tries to help, by exchanging a reasonable view of health for something technical and inaccessible to the uninitiated.[5]

Our understanding of the social determinants of health is perhaps the best modern articulation of the idea that health is also externally located.[6] Where you live, what your family is like, and how you make a living all have more impact on your life expectancy than your medical care. We recognise social factors as important, but still only insofar as they affect measurable or disease-based outcomes, as if these were the only things that mattered. Would we really tolerate damp, overcrowded accommodation if it didn't increase our cardiovascular risk? Going for a walk isn't healthy because it helps you get your ten thousand steps in, but because we are not built for sitting at a desk all day, and because the world we live in is *out there*, no matter how much time we spend online or immersed in our thoughts. Meeting up with friends is not a way of preventing mental health problems; it's just part of being human. Can we really expect to be healthy by any definition if we neglect these things?

Too much of what we do as doctors is inherently negative, trying to avoid or manage illness rather than helping people to live healthy lives. We often feel this when we see patients lost in a jungle of symptoms without any biomedical cause, who would probably benefit more from an examination of their life than another round of blood tests and referrals. Even when it's clear that someone's situation is making them ill, we sometimes still reluctantly prescribe in order to keep them going because the alternatives all seem worse, or because we're rarely in a position to do much else. And yet there are times too when we can be surprised by how *healthy* some people seem, in the sense of living their life well, despite the presence of long-term illness or disability: here too, what we see depends on whether we are looking in or looking out.[7] It's easy for doctors and patients alike to feel overwhelmed by everything they're dealing with, but there are sometimes grounds for hope, and ways through the jungle, which we can glimpse if we adjust our view.

References

1. Porter, Roy, *The Greatest Benefit to Mankind: A Medical History of Humanity from Antiquity to the Present*. Harper Collins, New York, 1997.

2. http://theguardian.com/society/2023/aug/18/new-blood-test-could-transform-treatment-for-children-with-fever

3. Alzheimer's: 'Promising' blood test for early stage of disease – BBC News https://www.bbc.co.uk/news/health-53567486

4. Galleri cancer test: What is it and who can get it? – BBC News https://www.bbc.co.uk/news/health-58544874

5. Illich, Ivan, *Medical Nemesis: The Expropriation of Health*. Calder Publishing, London, 1976.

6. Marmot, Michael, *The Health Gap*. Bloomsbury, London, 2016.

7. Rousseau MC, Pietra S, Nadji M, Billette de Villemeur T. Evaluation of Quality of Life in Complete Locked-in Syndrome Patients. *J Palliat Med*. 2013;16(11):1455–1458.

Living in the Third Age of Medicine

For as long as there have been people, there have been those who needed looking after, whether due to frailty, poverty, injury or sickness, and those who looked after them. Disease has been one misfortune among many, all with the same general remedy: summon what help you can and await events. Where societies have had the benefit of healers of one sort or another, they have certainly done their best to improve their patients' outlook, but a larger part of their function has been interpretive: to provide context and direct expectations during this wait, often with a kind of medical theatre, "amusing the patient while nature cures the disease."[1]

Doctors have always played their part in this, largely because for most of our history there hasn't been much else that we could do. Despite its shortcomings, however, this kind of medicine is inherently patient-centred, springing from an individual's worldview, values and concerns, and addressing the unique experience of their illness, and it is still the foundation for much of what we do today.

If this First Age of medicine was concerned with interpreting illness, the Second Age was all about treating it and grew out of the scientific revolution, leading over time to hygiene, antibiotics, organ transplants and gene therapy. This is the medicine we learned as undergraduates, based on recognising the symptoms and signs of disease and applying the appropriate treatment. It concerns itself with pathology more than people, who are seen as cases of a condition rather than individuals with their own story. It can at times be frightening and dehumanising, but is also highly effective: think of all the medical and surgical advances of the last century and imagine what life would be like without them.

DOI: 10.1201/9781003652045-24

In the First and Second Ages, medicine was transacted between individual patients and doctors at times of illness. The Third Age, in which we find ourselves currently, is associated with the development of a much bigger picture in which this is no longer the case. Instead, healthcare systems interact continuously with whole populations, blurring the boundary between health and illness.

This process is analogous to the idea in business of vertical integration.[2] A company manufacturing a product is part of a supply chain, in which it depends on others both further back in the chain, and further forward. In order to have something to sell, it first needs investment, raw materials, tools, premises and a trained workforce. In order to sell, it needs marketing, distribution, retail and customer support. As a company grows, it can become more efficient by taking on these roles itself, integrating in both directions with its supply chain.

In the United Kingdom, we see the National Health Service simply as a provider of healthcare, but it already shows a high degree of vertical integration. Inasmuch as the NHS is a part of the state apparatus, it is integrated with its finance through taxation, its workforce through government involvement in training, and its research and development through public funding of academia. Although at the retail end GP partnerships are technically independent contractors, they are in effect franchise-holders, and some are already employed directly. None of this is controversial, but it has profound implications for patients.

Patients are generally considered either beneficiaries or consumers of healthcare. Gradually and without realising it, however, they have also become a part of the supply chain. Their role has become to behave in such a way that the health service functions smoothly. In practical terms, this means accepting an emphasis on preventive care, screening and early proactive management of non-specific presentations to avoid their costly escalation.[3] We go along with this every time we initiate primary cardiovascular prevention or refer a patient for investigation because of a combination of demographics and everyday symptoms which may be associated with cancer. In this situation, we are no longer acting to cure a sick patient or to help them make sense of their experience; we are risk-managing them based on health-economic considerations.

Naturally, patients don't want to have strokes or cancer, but most of those who take cholesterol-lowering tablets or attend fast-track clinics do not benefit, and some come to harm. This kind of medicine places on both doctors and patients a heavy burden of responsibility for preventing sickness and death, while at the same time minimising any real sense of agency.

The population may have better measurable outcomes, but neither the doctor nor the patient is likely to notice the difference. Furthermore, if the only reason I am recommending statins this year is that they are cheaper than last year, the implication is that everyone ought to be on them if we could afford it, and that no one is healthy really.

Health is being redefined neither as a state of maximum wellbeing nor as the absence of disease, but as the lowest point on a curve representing the risk of any sort of adverse outcome. Most of these outcomes are clinical, but others, like unplanned hospitalisation or litigation, are not in principle bad for patients, but put an additional strain on the system. It is significant that since the COVID-19 pandemic it has become normal to talk about the need to prevent the NHS from becoming overwhelmed, as if the survival of the system were the main aim.[4] Granted, the health service can only benefit patients if it is functioning, and it is inevitable that an overstretched service will do this less well, but the change in emphasis suggests that we are now thinking in terms of managing a supply chain in which patients are just a part, and perhaps not the part they thought.

Patients connected to a healthcare system generate demographic, physiological and disease-related data which contribute to a dynamic picture of the health of the whole population. Analysis of these data can be used to plan services and conduct research, to fine-tune the system. Useful though this is, there is something disconcerting about the idea of people becoming not just patients, but mere data points, the end result of this particular supply chain, in the same way that we become the digital product whenever we use an internet search engine.[5]

The Third Age of medicine is at once the most benign and the most unsettling. We now have the organisational, medical and informatic tools to mitigate the effects of disease to an extraordinary degree. In order to use these tools to their full effect, however, we must submit to being constantly monitored and managed, and do more and more to safeguard our health despite knowing that we are unlikely to benefit directly, lest by getting it wrong we somehow break the machinery intended to care for us. In the words of CS Lewis, *Of all tyrannies, a tyranny sincerely exercised for the good of its victims may be the most oppressive.*[6]

Perhaps my reservations are not so much to do with practicalities, but with the principle. Given the choice, would we rather do our best to get on with life and not worry about our health, or do whatever it takes to avoid serious illness? As doctors, we can help our patients regardless of how they answer this question, but we must at least ensure that they understand it.

References

1. "The art of medicine consists in amusing the patient while nature cures the disease," attributed to Voltaire from the end of the 19th century, but probably apocryphal; earlier versions are generally anonymous, as in The Quarterly Journal of Science, Literature, and the Arts 1823: "'Physic,' says a foreign writer, "is the art of amusing..."' http://oxfordreference.com

2. Iliffe, Steve, *From General Practice to Primary Care: The Industrialization of Family Medicine*. Oxford University Press, Oxford, 2008.

3. McCartney, Margaret, *The Patient Paradox: Why Sexed-up Medicine is Bad for Your Health*. Pinter & Martin, London, 2012.

4. For a recent example, see NHS crisis: Health leaders raise alarm over 'overwhelmed' hospitals at No. 10 summit with Rishi Sunak (inews.co.uk) inews.co.uk/news/nhs-crisis-health-leaders-downing-street-rishi-sunak-forum-2070856

5. The idea that the consumer becomes the product can be traced to a 1973 video by Richard Serra and Carlota Fay Schoolman, which included the statement in relation to TV advertising, "It is the consumer who is consumed. You are the product of t.v." http://quoteinvestigator.com

6. Lewis CS, *God in the Dock: Essays on Theology and Ethics*. Erdmans, London, first published 1970.

Networks, Nodes and Equilibrium

On any given day, GPs diagnose and treat, listen, validate, interpret, advise, support and advocate. A large part of what we do, though, is indirect, by linking patients with various other parts of the healthcare system. When we prescribe, investigate or refer, we are asking a pharmacist, laboratory technician, radiographer or fellow-clinician to act on a patient's behalf, albeit in more or less specific ways. We function as a node connecting patients to a wider network.

If we think a bit more about what this network looks like, it makes sense to start with another node representing the patient, connected to ours, but also to others: informal health advisers, including friends and family; non-healthcare professionals, like teachers, social workers and probation officers; and directly accessible healthcare professionals, such as pharmacists, nurses, midwives and paramedics. All of these may effectively refer a patient to their GP, just as their GP may refer them to another professional with a more specialised role.

We can picture a model, then: on the left side are the patient and their connections, and on the right, the GP and theirs; the two halves are linked to each other through a single connection, that between patient and doctor. There is a flow from left to right, as, for example, when a grandparent's concern about a child prompts their parent to arrange a consultation at the surgery and agree on referral to a paediatrician, who might, in turn, arrange a dietetic assessment, and so on.

This is a reasonable model of the NHS a generation ago, with the relationship between a patient and their GP at the centre of the network. The ability to hold uncertainty and make shared decisions at this point moderates flow from left to right by preventing inappropriate medicalisation,

DOI: 10.1201/9781003652045-25

holding back the worried well and waving through the vulnerable. Since then, however, the number of GPs has fallen,[1] and the expectations of policy-makers have shifted. In particular, the drive to diagnose cancer earlier has, to some extent, made primary care a clearing house for patients with non-specific symptoms waiting to be investigated.

Between 2009/10 and 2019/20, GP referrals for suspected cancers increased by 163%, driving down the rate of positive diagnosis from 10.8% to 6.6%.[2] The recommended threshold for referral is a nominal 3% risk of having cancer,[3] however, implying that despite the huge increase in referrals, we should still be sending far more patients to secondary care than we are. Deliberately increasing traffic within the system and directing it through a narrowing channel seems a little like closing your eyes and putting your foot down when you see the lights change.

This has no doubt contributed to our current professional malaise, as well as causing a proliferation of actual and proposed work-arounds: secondary care services directly accessible by patients which create new connections between the two halves of the network, bypassing general practice. In theory, these allow patients to arrange their own care without needing to see a doctor, but, in practice, they also transfer the control in the system from the doctor–patient relationship to the various protocols that govern these new pathways. If you know how to access a service, you can self-refer, but you may just get a letter advising you that you don't meet the threshold to be taken on; those less able to negotiate this increasingly complex and rigid system inevitably lose out.

The management of uncertainty is likewise changing: rather than being buffered in general practice, it is now more likely to be cryogenically preserved in secondary care, through the prolonged follow-up of patients with incidental findings like lung nodules and mildly raised Prostate Specific Antigen levels.

At a time when the benefits arising from continuity of care in general practice have been well established,[4] demonstrating clearly the importance of the relationship between patients and their doctor, the network within which this relationship plays such a significant role is gradually being reconfigured to make it redundant. This may eventually result in a new equilibrium, in which GPs no longer regulate the wider network but become merely one node among many within it. It would be easy in this scenario to lament our loss of influence, although we might also find that instead of making an appointment just for us to pass them on to someone else, patients came to see us because they believed that we had something of value to offer them ourselves. I hope I get to see it!

References

1. Pressures in general practice data analysis (bma.org.uk) https://www.bma.org.uk/advice-and-support/nhs-delivery-and-workforce/pressures/pressures-in-general-practice-data-analysis

2. Early Diagnosis (shinyapps.io) https://crukcancerintelligence.shinyapps.io/Early Diagnosis/

3. Context | Suspected cancer: recognition and referral | Guidance | NICE https://www.nice.org.uk/guidance/ng12/chapter/Context

4. Pereira-Grey D, Sidaway-Lee K, White E, Thorne A, Evans P. Improving continuity: THE clinical challenge. *InnovAiT* 2016;9:10. https://doi.org/10.1177/175573 8016654504

Efficiency, Effectiveness, and Communities of Practice

The number of GP surgeries in the UK is falling, through either mergers or outright closures, and those that remain are becoming larger.[1] This growth in practice size is a significant change, for which I would like to suggest three potential explanations. The first is that once the number of practices closing in a given area exceeds the number opening, the only option for patients and staff is to join an existing one, so that the change merely reflects the ongoing pressures on general practice. The second is that larger practices may provide a better service, prompting those that can to grow, even at the expense of smaller neighbours. The third is that regardless of quality, larger practices may simply be better at surviving. More than one of these explanations might apply: practices do many different things, some of which are likely to work better on a larger or smaller scale, and all of which could affect their financial viability as well as the care they provide; and even in hard times, small differences between practices may allow some to stay open, while others close. The powers that be certainly seem to equate bigger with better, viewing Primary Care Networks (PCNs) of at least thirty thousand patients as optimal for the purposes of funding and service provision. Patients take the opposite view, with a negative correlation between size and satisfaction, and the highest level of satisfaction found in practices with a list size of less than ten thousand.[2] How can we make sense of both these views?

It is well recognised that businesses of different sizes have contrasting advantages. Larger ones tend to be associated with a higher degree of specialisation, more clearly defined structures and hierarchies, and economies of scale; smaller ones, with less role differentiation, a more flexible and cooperative structure, and greater agility. It is easy to see this reflected in

DOI: 10.1201/9781003652045-26

general practice. Larger surgeries will tend to experience more predictable demand, giving them the stability to provide specific services in areas like acute illness, musculoskeletal problems and mental ill health. They will be able to access funding for such services through their PCN and will be well-suited to adopting the multi-professional team model promoted by NHS England, with arm's-length initial contact followed by the allocation of patients to specific clinicians based on the nature of their problem.[3] Those working in smaller practices, on the other hand, will find it easier to maintain relationships with each other and with their patients, favouring a more collaborative and generalist way of working, and benefitting from greater personal continuity of care, although they will find it more difficult to pay for these things.[4] Perhaps we can characterise these two kinds of practice as representing either *efficiency* in providing a high volume of appointments or *effectiveness* in making each appointment count for more. As a practice grows, we can expect it to become more efficient, although there is likely to come a point, beyond which further gains in efficiency come at the expense of reduced effectiveness.

To see why this might be the case, it may help to consider the idea of a *community of practice*. The term describes a group of people working in pursuit of the same goals, using the same tools, and working out together what needs to be done and how to go about it.[4] Such a community relies on arrangements which maximise interactions between its members, including adjoining work spaces, communal areas, and rotas that guarantee overlapping work and break times. Its members are neither specialists with distinct roles, nor duplicates enacting a standard set of procedures, but colleagues, each bringing to the table their own experience and perspective. Whereas practitioners working in isolation follow national or international guidelines, communities of practice create their own *mindlines*, which fulfil a similar purpose, but are locally negotiated and owned, and sensitive to local contexts.[5] In this sense, communities of practice become specialised in dealing with their constituency rather than a particular problem.

Clinicians in a practice represent one such community, while administrators make up another, and patients have the potential to form a third. How well these three communities interact internally and with each other depends, at least partly, on the layout of a given surgery, including the reception, waiting room and adjacent consulting rooms, office space, and shared staff area. Even with an ideal layout, and taking into account the impact of remote working and patient access, the level of interaction needed for communities of practice to function effectively will only take place up to a certain size. Beyond this, a larger building containing signposted corridors and numbered doors to identical, hygienically optimised cubicles becomes conceptually more like a hospital, even if it contains GPs, inasmuch as it represents the privileging of process over meaningful personal interaction.

Economies of scale, and the ability to provide more specialised services in return for increased funding, will tend to favour a growth in practice size, while the requirements of interpersonal care and the communities of practice with which it is associated, probably mandate an upper limit to this. Given the current realities of general practice, however, it seems likeliest that we will simply see a continued shift towards larger and more efficient surgeries, providing ever-more appointments, but perhaps achieving less of what patients really need or want. Let us beware of seeking efficiency in isolation, and at the expense of effectiveness.

References

1. NHS Digital, General Practice Trends in the UK to 2017. https://digital.nhs.uk/data-and-information/areas-of-interest/workforce/technical-steering-committee-tsc/technical-steering-committee-tsc-archive

2. Edwards, PJ. Bigger Practices Are Associated with Decreased Patient Satisfaction and Perceptions of Access. *Br J Gen Pract* 2022;72(722):420–421. https://doi.org/10.3399/bjgp22X720521

3. NHS England, Modern General Practice Model https://england.nhs.uk/gp/national-general-practice-improvement-programme/modern-general-practice-model/

4. Gray DP, Sidaway-Lee K, Whitaker P, Evans P. Adverse Effects for Patients In Big Group Practices. *Br J Gen Pract* 2022;72(724):518. https://doi.org/10.3399/bjgp22X720989

5. Gabbay John and Le May Andrée, *Practice-based Evidence for Healthcare: Clinical Mindlines*. Routledge, Abingdon and New York, 2011.

6. Wenger Etienne, *Communities of Practice: Learning, Meaning, and Identity*. Cambridge University Press, Cambridge, 1998.

Imagining the Future

You may not consider yourself a fan of science fiction, but we are all travellers in time, moving together into the future at the same steady pace. The fact that we think about *the future* as distinct from the present acknowledges that we expect it to be different: distance travelled equals rate of change multiplied by time, and even within a professional lifetime, we are likely to end up a long way from where we started. *The past is a foreign country: they do things differently there*, but we could say the same of the future.[1]

Of course, the future has a habit of becoming the present, and then the past. Mary Shelley, Jules Verne and H.G. Wells all speculated about what might lie beyond a horizon which we passed long ago. Today's cutting edge, the preserve of the privileged few, will be taken for granted by our children. As William Gibson put it, *The future's already here: it's just not evenly distributed.*[2]

Advances in science and technology have always gone together with social change, from the development of the crossbow that allowed a commoner to bring down a knight on horseback, to the migration of labourers into the cities during the industrial revolution. The details of how this works out in practice, though, can be unpredictable. It is hardly surprising that micro-processors become more powerful and portable as technology progresses, but isn't it interesting that we've ended up with the telephone as the predominant form of personal computer, and that we use ours so much to access social media? Any discussion of what our society will look like in fifty or a hundred years' time is likely to be dominated by climate change, overpopulation and ageing, but can we imagine the details?

The place of Medicine in our imagined future, science fiction, tends to be defined by technology. In the original 1960s TV series *Star Trek*, Dr McCoy

DOI: 10.1201/9781003652045-27

used a medical tricorder in place of a stethoscope, but he was still recognisable as a curmudgeonly doctor. More often, medics are portrayed as faceless and amoral, technicians operating the miracle machines that extend life, heal and enhance. They are doers, but not talkers or listeners. In the 2013 film *Elysium*, the machinery can be operated by anyone, removing the need for doctors altogether.

Some visions of the future are darker. In William Gibson's cyberpunk novels the body is weaponised and booby-trapped, and the central nervous system becomes at times little more than a user interface connected to the matrix of cyberspace. Cyborgs, people altered by technology to the point where they lose their humanity, are darker still, the modern equivalent of the medieval Dr Faustus, who sold his soul to the devil in return for magical power.

Andrew Niccol's 1997 film *Gattaca* is more hopeful. In a future society peopled by the *valid*, genetically selected to have the best chance of health and success, and the *invalid*, born the old-fashioned way, the conclusion is that a flawed individual can still succeed against the odds. Indeed, we are left to reflect that in a system built on reason and control, it is our capacity for irrationality and unpredictability that somehow defines us as human. Our technology lets us change the world according to our needs and preferences, but a part of us still longs to be *au naturel* and free of the artificial carapace we have made for ourselves. We live in cities but dream of the countryside, design intelligent robots and worry that one day they will turn against us.

As in science fiction, so in medicine there is a constant tension between the technological and the human, what is possible and what is desirable. Are we to measure health purely in terms of years lived and diseases avoided, or something less tangible but more meaningful? We are certainly getting very good at the former. There is a tension, though, and how that tension is sustained or resolved will have a huge impact on what General Practice looks like for us and for our patients as we see the future become more evenly distributed. If we want a future that we can live with, we need to start imagining what it looks like now.

References

1. Hartley LP, *The Go-Between*, first published by Hamish Hamilton, London, 1953.

2. Aphorism expressed variously by William Gibson, quoted in this form on the jacket of *Distrust That Particular Flavour: encounters with a future that's already here*, Penguin, New York, 2012.

Not Just a Theory?

Transcript begins

Newshound:	Thanks for agreeing to see me, doctor...
Subject:	John, it's just John these days. I appreciate your making the trip. Did anyone try to stop you?
Newshound:	No, I don't think so, not unless you count the sheep in the lane.
Subject:	Are you being funny? I thought you were serious about doing this interview.
Newshound:	Hey, no offence, doc, it's just a little out of the way, you know?
Subject:	Sure, sorry, I'm a bit jumpy with everything that's happened. Do you want to make a start?
Newshound:	That would be great. I'm a bit slower with the old pen and paper, but you said no tech.
Subject:	Thanks. Everyone laughs when you start talking about conspiracies, but they happen all the time: I'll get my mate to approve your extension if you can sort out my tax problem. Lovely yacht, chief, I'll have a word with the minister about fast-tracking your new wonder-drug, just make sure those trial data don't get into the official record...
Newshound:	You're talking about what you refer to as the medical-pharmaceutical-academic-fundraising complex now. Not exactly catchy, is it?

DOI: 10.1201/9781003652045-28

Subject:	Course not, too many players, blooming circus. The military-industrial complex was a joke by comparison. How much money gets spent on the military these days, and how much on health? During the Cold War, everyone was scared of the Russians, now it's disease. They use our fear to control us, to distract us from the real issues and make money on the side.
Newshound:	The real issues?
Subject:	Social determinants of health, mate: if you want to be healthy, don't bother about your Bupa cover, just make sure you grow up in the right part of town with a full complement of parents, get a decent education, proper job, nice house, pension. That's the stuff that needs looking at. We're living longer than ever, we're healthier than ever, and all you ever hear is that we're going to hell in a handbag because you can't get an appointment with your GP and the hospitals are full.
Newshound:	Don't you think the NHS is in crisis then?
Subject:	If you get hammered and wrap your Mondeo around a tree, then sure, you've got a crisis, but you can hardly blame the car.
Newshound:	You're saying you think the Health Service has been mismanaged?
Subject:	Mismanaged my foot. They know what they're doing. First you tell everyone they're in danger from something really nasty. Next, when people are good and worried, you make it harder for them to see a doctor and put pictures on the news of patients on trollies in hospital corridors and nurses on strike until they start demanding better services, and then you can reluctantly push up taxes to pay for it all. Supply and demand, right?
Newshound:	Isn't that a bit cynical?
Subject:	How else do you explain wage stagnation, capping medical school places and micromanaging primary care? Nobody sane would think any of that stuff would actually help. Whoever thought of charging hospital staff for parking was a blooming genius!
Newshound:	So what's the answer then?

Subject:	Stop trying to frighten everyone and let them get on with life. Bottom line: we all die eventually, so don't worry about it, make the most of your life and try to leave the world a better place for your kids when you're done. If you're sick, go and see a doctor, but don't make yourself sick taking pills and getting scanned every five minutes because there's a small chance you've got something serious, or might have ten years down the line. Treat people like adults and they'll start looking after themselves better too.
Newshound:	And if people don't listen?
Subject:	Direct action. Start with the academics, then Big Pharma. Sabotage the scanners. Once people see they don't need it all, they'll feel much better.
Newshound:	That's fighting talk. I take it the establishment doesn't approve.
Subject:	That's how I ended up out here, off the grid: no one wants a doctor who tells patients they're okay and stands up to the system. I got tired of checking my home for bugs and my car for bombs. One day people will get it, and I'll be ready.
Newshound:	Great stuff, John, gotta shoot now but I've got what I need. I'll send you a copy of the interview before it goes to press.
Subject:	Thanks, I just want to help make things better.
...	
Newshound:	War-dog, this is Newshound, over.
War-dog:	Go ahead, Newshound, over.
Newshound:	War-dog, subject is confirmed, you are cleared to engage, over.
War-dog:	Wilco, over.
Newshound:	Roger, out.

Transcript ends.

Diverging at the Horizon*

Train-tracks approaching the horizon appear to converge, although in reality, they remain equidistant. UK General Practice finds itself on a train journey along tracks which seem to do the opposite: the further down the line we look, the more they diverge. Should we disembark at the earliest opportunity before disaster strikes, or sit tight and see what happens? Perhaps it's just an illusion, and we can return to our book or look out of the window, untroubled by horizon-anxiety.

One of our rails represents a programme with which perhaps few of us feel totally comfortable, but which has gradually become a part of day-to-day practice. Its emphasis is on proactive, preventive care, and it is inherently risk-averse. Its implicit aspiration is to eliminate disease, and the tools used to achieve this are largely technological and process-based, with an army of generic clinicians implementing approved care pathways, which lead to a variety of diagnostic procedures. This is healthcare at scale, transacted between the citizen and the system on behalf of the people at large, and its motto is *one missed case is one case too many*. Its dark side is the creeping medicalisation of daily life, and the creation of an informer-state in which every symptom must be reported to the authorities. It sees health as a property of populations, for which individuals are expected to give up their freedom not to worry, and do their civic duty.

The other rail is one that feels more friendly and familiar, if at times a little quaint. It puts the doctor–patient relationship at the centre of care,

---

* An earlier version of this piece was published as: Hoban B. Diverging at the horizon. *Br J Gen Pract*. 2024 Apr 25;74(742):215. doi: 10.3399/bjgp24X737217. PMID: 38664048; PMCID: PMC11060824.

DOI: 10.1201/9781003652045-29

and it focuses on the individual and their concerns. Its aim is to enable the rest of life, and it therefore sees the significance of a given symptom as much in terms of its impact on a patient's function as the percentage chance that it might be caused by a cancer. According to this approach, a good patient is one who does their best to get on with life, and a good doctor is one who is available when needed. It recognises death and disease as inevitable and does little to challenge the societal factors that distribute ill health so unevenly. It accepts much, but helps where it can – more of a benevolent grandparent than an omnipotent dictator.

We are travelling over bumpy ground. The introduction of the Additional Roles Reimbursement Scheme illustrates both the need to expand the primary care workforce and the challenges inherent in combining different professional cultures in a single workplace. Rather than dividing up our workload on the basis of who else can do it – musculoskeletal cases for physios, psychological problems for mental health practitioners, medication reviews for pharmacists – when the whole point of our role is generalism, why not look instead at where it comes from? Those driving NHS policy place a high value on cardiovascular risk reduction and earlier cancer diagnosis across the population, and these have become tangled up with the normal process of looking after patients, who, by and large, want to see their doctor about things that matter more to them personally. The answer to the question "Am I okay, doc?" is not expressed in numbers.

As we rattle through our busy days, our train still rests on both these rails, and often rocks from one side to the other within a given consultation. The dearth of doctors in primary care, and the need for them to supervise non-medical staff at the expense of their own clinical work, may push us towards a more transactional kind of medicine. On the other hand, a growing awareness of the benefits of personal care may yet pull us back towards something more easily recognisable as General Practice. Perhaps we will just continue on our journey with the same tensions that exist now, but it's not difficult to imagine a future parting of the ways, with a new national service offering risk-based screening and preventive medicine, while GPs focus on caring for those who feel unwell. It may be that our bumpy train journey will end, not in disaster, but at a shiny new terminal, where we can board one of two monorails heading in different directions. I know which one I'll be riding.

Health Perception

It has been observed that people living in more affluent parts of the world with better healthcare and less disease tend to have a lower view of their health than people in poorer areas, where disease is more prevalent and healthcare less well-developed.[1] Bizarre as this is, it may shine a light on some of our current difficulties in the National Health Service.

For many globally today, as in previous generations in the UK, high maternal and infant mortality, an inadequate diet, fatal infectious diseases, violence and unsafe working and living conditions are facts of life. If you want to be healthier, the solution may not be within reach at the moment, but it isn't complicated: find a reliable source of income or other help that will allow you to eat nutritious food, drink clean water and live somewhere safe, with accessible healthcare for when you are ill, having children or in need of contraception. The factors limiting your health are all external, and a healthier life is an aspiration, something to move towards in a known direction. It isn't easy, but it makes sense.

In today's UK, life by any objective measure is longer, safer and less limited by disease than ever before. Health is still largely socially determined, but for most people this is more about the impact of inequalities inherent in an affluent society than any absolute need: we are more concerned about childhood obesity than protein-energy malnutrition, scurvy or rickets.[2] Most of the patients we see are not in immediate danger: our role is usually to consider the possibility of a serious underlying cause of their symptoms, or to try to prevent serious illness in the future. We do this by investigating and by managing risk factors, acknowledging that while we are reducing the burden of disease in the population as a whole, the vast majority of individuals don't benefit directly.

DOI: 10.1201/9781003652045-30

For most of us, health has become something we're used to having, but also something that we fear disproportionately to lose; as with money, we reckon the value of our losses more highly than what we never had to begin with.[3] The threats to our health are more subtle and located within our own body now: disease is seen as something that could come at any moment with little or no warning, and from any direction. If our grandparents with their aspirations of a healthier life resembled sailors making their way in an open boat to a distant harbour, we are more like passengers on a luxury yacht, becalmed and waiting for Leviathan to strike. Patients and doctors are responsible for being vigilant, reporting anything unexpected and taking what precautions they can, even though it may not help them. We have come to accept health scares as the price of health.

We are therefore healthier than people elsewhere and in the past, but only at the cost of much introspection, hyper-vigilance, and learned helplessness,[4] or, in the words of Arthur Frank, *embodied paranoia*.[5] We are expending huge efforts to add further gains still, pushing asymptotically towards a vision of perfect health, but it is worth wondering whether we would be able to enjoy it if we ever got there. Samuel Butler's Victorian satire *Erewhon* imagines a country in which everyone is beautiful, strong and robustly healthy, but in which illness is viewed as a moral failing and punished severely. We can certainly try to improve our patients' health by investigating their symptoms and managing their risk of disease, but perhaps it's time to ask ourselves whether there are also times when we would be helping them more by encouraging a greater confidence in the health they have already.

References

1. Sen A. Health: Perception versus Observation. *BMJ* 2002;324:860–861.

2. Marmot Michael, *The Health Gap: The Challenge of An Unequal World*. Bloomsbury, London, 2016.

3. Kahneman Daniel, *Thinking, Fast and Slow*. Penguin, New York, 2012.

4. Illich Ivan, *Limits to Medicine: Medical Nemesis – The Expropriation of Health*. Marion Boyars, London, 1976.

5. Frank Arthur, *The Wounded Storyteller*. 2nd Ed. University of Chicago Press, Chicago, 2013.

HOW THE SYSTEM WORKS

Wagging the Dog*

The time-honoured reward for a job well done is more jobs to do well, and fewer resources with which to do them. On this basis, GPs have been well rewarded over the years. Complaints about workload, especially the kind that represents poor use of our time, are nothing new, although it feels as if there has been more to complain about for a while. The inappropriate transfer of work from secondary care, in particular, is a well-recognised problem which seems difficult to address.[1, 2]

Medical care of any kind inevitably generates lists of jobs, some of which are straightforward and can be done by anyone, such as looking up blood results at the end of the day, and others that require a more detailed knowledge of the patient and their situation. Even simple tasks can only be delegated successfully, however, if the working relationship between the donor and recipient allows it: at the most basic level, a senior transfers work to a junior on the basis that they also take responsibility for the junior's actions; and one colleague hands over jobs to another at the end of a shift today on the basis of quid pro quo tomorrow. The relationship between primary and secondary care involves its own kind of reciprocity, although it is perhaps more like that between patients and GPs.[3]

Just as the ideas, concerns and expectations of the patient ought usually to set the agenda in a consultation, so those of the general practitioner are the natural starting point for what happens in secondary care. This doesn't always mean that one simply makes work for the other: it is reasonable for a GP to advise patients how to look after themselves, and for a specialist to advise us what we can do to help someone we have referred. The key in

* An earlier version of this piece was published as: Hoban B. Wagging the dog. *Br J Gen Pract*. 2024 Aug 29;74(746):421. doi: 10.3399/bjgp24X739353. PMID: 39209710; PMCID: PMC11349376.

DOI: 10.1201/9781003652045-31

both cases is that the advice meets an agreed need and falls within the recipient's normal sphere: if a patient is concerned about cardiovascular disease, I can ask them to arrange a blood test to measure their cholesterol level, but not a coronary CT. If a hospital colleague asks me to review someone's analgesia following an admission, I'd be happy to, but if they want to hand over their pre-discharge task list, I'll be handing it back.

What we consider reasonable for patients or GPs to do is, of course, constantly changing. Technologies like pulse oximetry and interstitial glucose monitoring that originate in secondary care are passed on to general practice and soon find their way into popular use without affecting the relationships between hospital and surgery, or doctor and patient. At the same time, however, there has been a much more fundamental change in our healthcare system that affects the flow of work, and the relationships, within it.

It is no longer self-evidently true that the purpose of the system is to safeguard the health of individual patients. Instead, these individuals are increasingly expected to act in a way that safeguards the health of the population at large – by attending appointments, undergoing investigations, and taking medication – even though they are unlikely to benefit themselves. By degrees, and without discussion, the patient's role has changed from actively setting a personal agenda for their care to passively accepting a medical agenda set by experts and politicians. In this inverted world, the transfer of work from secondary to primary care mirrors the transfer of responsibility from the system to its users. The traditional intermediary role of general practice between patients and the wider health service has changed too, although it is increasingly bypassed by screening programmes, community specialty teams, and hospital electronic record platforms: we now act less to enable patients to access the system when they need to, and more to enable the system to access patients whenever "best practice" requires it.

Perhaps the clearest illustration of this shift is the changing balance of consultant and GP numbers in the NHS. Seventy years ago, there were nearly three times as many GPs as consultants. Both groups grew steadily until the mid-1990s, although the gap between them was narrowing; since then, GP growth has been flatlining while the increase in consultant numbers has accelerated and there are now more than twice as many Full-Time Equivalent consultants as GPs.[4-6] The bigger picture when we consider "work-dumping" is therefore not that individual hospital practitioners are behaving unreasonably, but that the system as a whole now favours a secondary care way of working, which meshes poorly with our own approach. While this may feel professionally threatening to us, the larger issue is that the medical establishment, which prioritises its own agenda, is taking from patients the ability to decide for themselves what it means to be healthy: the tail is wagging the dog.

The new Secretary of State for Health and Social Care has promised to address the disparity in funding between primary and secondary care. Let us hope that we end up not just with more money, but with a more balanced system overall, for the sake of our patients as well as our workload.

References

1. Price A, Majeed, A. Improving How Secondary Care and General Practice in England Work Together: Requirements in the NHS Standard Contract. *J R Soc Med* 2018;111(2):42–46. https://doi.org/10.1177/0141076817738504

2. Mughal Z, Maharjan R. Cross-sectional Analysis of Hospital Tasks Handed Over to General Practitioners: Workload Delegation or Dumping? *Postgrad Med J* July 2022;98(1161):e14. https://doi.org/10.1136/postgradmedj-2020-139641

3. Khan N. Workload transfer in the NHS: The Great British Dump – BJGP Life 8 December 2023.

4. Moberly, T. Data Chart: Consultant Numbers Have Doubled Over the Past 20 Years, *BMJ* 2017;359:j4726 https://doi.org/10.1136/bmj.j4726

5. NHS medical staffing data analysis (bma.org.uk) https://www.bma.org.uk/advice-and-support/nhs-delivery-and-workforce/workforce/nhs-medical-staffing-data-analysis

6. Pressures in general practice data analysis (bma.org.uk) https://www.bma.org.uk/advice-and-support/nhs-delivery-and-workforce/pressures/pressures-in-general-practice-data-analysis

Cautionary Tales*

Everyone loves a good story. Stories entertain us, but, on a deeper level, they also help us make sense of our experience; they are cultural vectors, transmitting the values and wisdom of one generation to the next. The proper use of power is a common theme in traditional tales: secret knowledge, wealth or authority can all be forces for good, but they are tools to be held lightly and applied with care in case of unintended consequences.

The sorcerer's apprentice popularised by Disney uses magic to do the cleaning, but ends up making a mess because he lacks his master's authority over the spirits he has summoned.[1] In the tale of the Golem, a rabbi animates a clay figure by inscribing on its head the name of God, but loses control of it after presuming to use its strength for profane ends.[2] Mary Shelley's obsessive scientist Victor Frankenstein builds an artificial human without first considering how to meet its human needs: the creature only becomes a monster because of Frankenstein's monstrous neglect.[3]

Neither does restraint in the use of power come easily to us in more mundane situations. Madeleine Albright, United States Secretary of State from 1997 to 2001, reportedly asked: "What's the point of having this superb military... if we can't use it?"[4] An armed force deployed to project power must use that power to some purpose, even one to which it is ill-suited, and its mission easily creeps.[5] We see something similar in the story of modern medicine.

Historically, medicine has provided a framework within which people who are sick can understand what is happening to them, know how to respond, and receive care from others. Doctors have generally lacked the

* An earlier version of this piece was published as: Hoban B. Cautionary tales. *Br J Gen Pract*. 2024 Jul 25;74(745):366. doi: 10.3399/bjgp24X738993. PMID: 39054100; PMCID: PMC11299673.

DOI: 10.1201/9781003652045-32

means to influence the outcome of an illness, but through their presence at the bedside and the comforting structure of a regime of treatment, they have perhaps made it a little easier for everyone to await events. Our focus has been less on fighting disease and more on helping people bear it.

This has changed radically within the last few hundred years, with the flourishing of biomedical science and the development of safe surgical treatment, effective drugs, and laboratory and radiological investigations that expose to us the workings of the living body as never before. We have collectively become so powerful that it is becoming difficult to accept that there are limits to what we can know or do. When someone is unwell, we expect to be able to diagnose and treat them promptly, and it no longer feels simply unfortunate when we cannot, but somehow wrong, an affront to our mastery over disease. Biomedicine has become such an accepted paradigm that, against a background of cultural ambivalence towards political or religious authority, it is now our default model for understanding problems that have consequences for health, like obesity or gang violence, even though they are not themselves diseases.[6, 7] In fact, we now concern ourselves largely with people who are not unwell in the usual sense at all, managing risk factors to prevent disease or identifying and treating it at the earliest possible stage. On one level this makes good sense, and we accept unquestioningly the idea that prevention is better than cure. On another, however, it represents a significant development in our story.

If medicine was previously framed interpersonally and socially, and geared towards the successful negotiation of ill health, we see it now more as a quest to eliminate disease through the application of scientific power. The benefits of this quest include our ability to treat conditions which, not long ago, would have been fatal, but the unintended consequences are widespread health-related anxiety and a paradoxical growth in the number of those who consider themselves unwell. We have become so preoccupied with our struggle against disease that we are in danger of neglecting these people, whom we have persuaded to become patients without enabling them to bear it well.[8]

If there is wisdom to be gained from stories, it is surely that we should take care not to let our power for good corrupt our good intentions. Medicine was, and always should be, primarily about looking after people, not just fixing parts of them. Rather than pursuing ever more power over disease, we should perhaps aim to use the power we already have to help people live their lives well.[9] It is, after all, the apprentice in the tale who looses the spirits, but the master who reins them in.

References

1. von Goethe JW, *Der Zauberlehrling*, 1797.

2. Deutsch A, *The Golem, Isaac Bashevis Singer*, André Deutsch, London, 1982.

3. Shelley Mary, *Frankenstein; or, The Modern Prometheus*. Lackington, Hughes, Harding, Mavor & Jones, London, 1818.

4. My American Journey, Colin Powell with Jospeh E Persico, Ballantine, 2003.

5. Smith Rupert, *The Utility of Force: The Art of War in the Modern World*. Penguin, 2006.

6. Preventing serious violence: summary – GOV.UK. http://gov.uk/government/publications/preventing-serious-violence-a-multi-agency-approach/preventing-serious-violence-summary

7. Wade DT, Halligan PW. Do Biomedical Models of Illness Make for Good Healthcare Systems? *BMJ* 2004;329:1398–1401.

8. Marinker M. Why Make People Patients? *J Med Ethics*, 1975;1:81–84.

9. Kleinman A. Catastrophe and Caregiving: The Failure of Medicine as an Art. *Lancet*. 2008;371:22–23.

A Poisoned Chalice?

I have to confess to mixed feelings on hearing that GPs will be invited to refer patients directly for radiological investigation of symptoms possibly due to cancer.[1] If you have cancer, it's usually better for it to be diagnosed early, and if poor GP access to imaging prevents this, then the change is welcome. Perhaps it's not quite that simple, though. Firstly, we're already in a position to investigate anyone with at least a 3% risk of having cancer by referring them to a fast-track outpatient service: the obvious conclusion is that we're being encouraged to lower the threshold for investigation beyond this. If we accept that clinically obvious tumours are relatively rare and may be too advanced for treatment to be successful, then it certainly makes sense to look for those at an earlier stage, presenting with milder and more non-specific symptoms. The problem, of course, is that mild and non-specific symptoms are widespread in the general population, so the Number Needed to Scan would be large.[2] If seeing patients once and referring them for imaging means they don't need to keep coming back for review, then early investigation offers advantages to busy GPs and busy patients alike, but, given the tendency of any test to throw up results of unclear significance, wouldn't we simply be delegating the management of uncertainty *en masse* to radiologists?

The subtext is also that general practice is just an outpost of hospital medicine, in which each symptom is linked by an invisible thread to a disease, as if the only purpose of listening to patients were to grasp this thread and follow it back to its origin. The Commons Health and Social Care Committee has cottoned on to the fact that continuity of care is a good

DOI: 10.1201/9781003652045-33

thing because it's associated with better outcomes like early diagnosis, and the level of continuity in a practice may one day be monitored alongside cervical smear uptake.[3] In this case we face the prospect of being held simultaneously over the barrels of biomedical efficiency and relational care.

The point of relational care, though, is surely not just that it is a more efficient way of diagnosing disease, but that it engages with both the humanity and the nebulousness of so many of our encounters with patients. The outcome of looking after people is sometimes just that they were looked after. In the same way as medicines have long been recognised to have a context-dependent effect irrespective of their active ingredients, so a certain amount of our activity is symbolic, communicating an important message: I am doing something for you because you are a person, just as I am a person, and it's my privilege to help you. We often inadvertently communicate other messages too: *the world is a terrifying place in which disease and death are never far away, but by being sufficiently vigilant and persistent, it's possible to avoid both; your story may seem meaningful to you, but its only value lies in the diagnostic clues it contains, which you are unqualified to interpret; even though I am a doctor, I can't make sense of what you're telling me, so you're probably lying.* We regularly see patients who have had a huge amount of medical input, without ever having felt *helped*.

We have reached a point where statistical analysis of aggregated patient data allows us to risk-manage individuals who would never consider themselves ill, such that the only well people may end up being those who haven't yet been sufficiently investigated.[4] Do we prioritise the ever-earlier diagnosis of disease, or the needs of patients looking for help to navigate the uncertainties of life and make sense of their personal experience of illness? Nobody wants to die of cancer, but should we expect patients to trust a faceless system which values only the length of their life rather than its significance? On one level, Medicine always fails; death is inevitable. There is another level, though, on which general practice, like palliative care, can always help despite this.

Open-access scans may help GPs work more effectively, but let's be wary of drinking too deeply from this cup.

References

1. All GPs to receive direct access to cancer tests – BBC News. https://www.bbc.co.uk/news/health-63642448

2. McAteer A, Elliott A, Hannaford P. Ascertaining the Size of the Symptom Iceberg in a UK-wide Community-based Survey. *BJGP* 2011. https://doi.org/10.3399/bjgp11X548910

3. *The Future of General Practice.* https://committees.parliament.uk/publications/30383/documents/176291/default/

4. Meador CK. The Last Well Person. *NEJM* 1994;330:440–441. https://doi.org/10.1056/NEJM199402103300618

The Deal

The doctor stands waiting, shivering in the July sunshine at a country crossroads a long way from home. The electric vehicle parked on the verge has managed the journey well despite all his range anxiety, and it turns out that roads outside the capital do appear on satellite navigation systems. He is wearing his second-best suit, hoping to give the impression of not trying too hard, but he is worried that after all he may be out of his depth. His partners know that he is away on a practice development activity, but he hasn't gone into detail with them, just in case it comes to nothing. You know how these things can be.

The dog-walker is irritating. She came out of the woods a couple of minutes ago with something on a lead that frankly looks like it would be more at home in Chelsea than out in the middle of wherever-it-is-shire. The dog yaps at his car while she stands there looking totally relaxed and – no, please – as if she is about to talk to him. Maybe this was all a mistake.

"You look a little lost, if you don't mind my saying so," she says.

"Thank you, I'm meeting someone, it's fine," he replies, forcing a little confidence into his voice.

"Yes, I see, although I wonder how well you know them."

Her comment is unexpected, and he experiences a sudden mix of confusion, annoyance and curiosity. His appraiser has encouraged him to cultivate a greater awareness of his emotional states during the consultation, and he thinks there might be something in it. He realises that despite all his preparation, he genuinely has no idea whom he is supposed to be meeting, and turns to look at this dog-walker more closely. She is casually dressed,

DOI: 10.1201/9781003652045-34

but in a way that still oozes money, above-average height, slim, must be in her fifties, although there is something older about her eyes, and a half-smile that suggests she is waiting for him to catch up, or perhaps a cat playing with a mouse. The penny drops.

"I'm so sorry, I'm Doctor –"

"I know, please don't worry. I'm not what most people expect, am I? No horns, no tail: I hope it's not too disappointing. You want something – everyone does – and you're hoping to make a deal."

"Yes, exactly! It's all been so difficult, what with the Quality and Outcomes Framework, the pandemic, the Primary Care Networks, having to supervise all those extra clinicians, and patients just won't look after themselves…" He realises that he has left his notes in the car and makes himself focus on his audience. She is just tying a knot in one of those disgusting plastic bags people collect dog mess in and then leave lying around anyway. She puts it into an expensive-looking tote and gives him her full attention in a way that instantly cuts him short. He registers a vague heaviness in the centre of his chest.

"Spare me the pitch. You are a failure. You find work frustrating but can't afford to retire, you think of yourself as a businessman but don't have the guts to push through your ideas, and you tell yourself that you want to help people, when really, you just want them to like you. You have nothing to offer me in return for saving your bacon except your cooperation. Fortunately for you, I like a little project." As he hears this, the doctor knows that it's all true, but can't help thinking of himself as a rasher of bacon, and suppresses a shudder. The woman is smiling, and he notices her perfect teeth.

"I have decided to devote my considerable resources to your case. We will need to start with your staff, whose attitude is recklessly unprofessional. There will be no more small-talk at reception or bending of rules for patients, who for the sake of clarity will be referred to as *units*. Those representing an unfavourable balance of costs and benefits will find that their relationship with the practice has irretrievably broken down and will be able to re-register elsewhere, while the rest will need to be properly motivated to ensure optimal compliance with your programme of preventive healthcare measures. A certain level of ambient fear works well: death and disease can be so *ugly* and I have some terrific ideas for your waiting room slide show. You will be able to grow your practice list through a proactive and robustly open-minded approach to prescribing opioids and benzodiazepines, and any units not fully engaged with the direction of travel of the business will find themselves suddenly resembling a cold turkey. Those fortunate enough to have skin tags will present themselves for quarterly minor surgery unless they want to end up at the back of the queue the next time HRT is hard to come by. Naturally, you will be far too busy managing this beacon of productivity to see any patients yourself, but will be in an excellent position to mentor the salaried doctors I shall be sending your way, whose unfortunate habits might make it difficult for them to secure employment elsewhere, and who will be more than happy with a minimum wage and the benefit of your discretion. I foresee a healthy practice, with excellent outcomes and optimal QOF scores. Can you feel the weight of my argument?"

The doctor is aware that the heaviness in his chest is both growing and spreading to his left arm. His head swims as he tries to keep track of a rapid succession of emotions – excitement, horror and fear – and he knows that his discomfort must be obvious. He sees that the woman's smile has grown too, however, and that she is showing more of those perfect teeth than seems strictly necessary. He reflects that, on balance, this was not a good idea. She extends her hand.

"Do we have a deal?"

PART III

How We Look after Patients

Everyone entering general practice is soon confronted with the reality that those certainties which we learned at medical school, however important, only represent a part of what we deal with every day in our surgeries. No matter how diligently we apply the biomedical model to contain our patients' symptoms, they still regularly spill over its sides, defying diagnosis or treatment; we cut off one problem's head, and, hydra-like, another two grow in its place. Quite apart from the challenge of dealing with our patients' expectations, we must also manage those of our paymasters, who are more interested in blood pressure than either backache or heartache, and of those absent third parties – a mother-in-law, neighbour or osteopath – whose advice sometimes carries more weight than our own. It can feel difficult to find the time to be patient-centred and relational on top of all this!

There is another side to this unsettling discovery, though, which more than compensates for it: we do not have to know, or fix, everything, and we do not have to do anything on our own; our patients are, for the most part, willing allies in their care, even if they sometimes disagree with us on particulars. A successful doctor–patient relationship is therefore not a negotiable extra, but the indispensable engine of effective practice.

Relationships are, at the most basic level, about the way two people manage the distance between them. Where there is no distance at all, there is no need for a relationship, and where the distance is too large, there can be none. The gap between doctor and patient is defined by many factors, including knowledge, perspective, language and values. If we accept that medicine is an uncertain business, and that it is the patient's concerns that

DOI: 10.1201/9781003652045-35

define the aims of the consultation, it becomes clear that a successful out-come depends not just on our medical skills, but just as much on how we bridge this gap. We must learn to foster rapport, trust and goodwill; to negotiate ambiguity and help people make sense of their experience; and, finally, to give them the confidence either to keep going through difficult times or pick themselves up again when they have fallen.

These things are not innate; we all learn interpersonal skills one way or another, and each appointment or phone call is an opportunity to practise. It may be that the most important lessons for us are, first of all, that this is worthwhile, and secondly, that the gap between us is smaller than we think: however different we are from our patients, we still have much in common with them. We may be doctors treating strangers, but we are all people first.

Heroes with Bifocals

We were all NHS heroes during the pandemic, at least officially. The story has moved on, however, and I suspect that most GPs feel at least an occasional heroism deficit in their day-to-day work. It may be heartening during these dark moments to consider that a doctor's career is a manifestation of a common narrative archetype known as The Hero's Journey.[1]

The young hero starts his or her journey at home, in many ways unremarkable, but with an inner spark that sets them aside from their peers. Through the conspiring of circumstances or the appearance of a mysterious elder, they experience the call to go to a distant land on a perilous quest that promises great rewards. The call may be resisted or put off for a time, but eventually the hero sets off, arriving after preliminary adventures at the edge of a gloomy swamp, cave, or other chthonic location. There, they must face a series of tests and trials before claiming the prize: a treasure, magical elixir, or some secret and powerful knowledge. The hero returns home to share this prize with a grateful world, but is forever changed by their quest, which separates them from the rest of humanity.

We see in the hero's journey the bones of a host of different fictional stories, as well as our own. We leave our old life behind to go to medical school. Like other students, we have fun and we learn, but sooner or later we find ourselves in the more primal surroundings of the dissecting room, the hospital ward or the mortuary, the sombre cave where we are confronted by death, disease and decay. We start to look at people as patients, their bodies as complex machines whose cogs and levers we learn to manipulate in the treatment of illness. We gradually pass through medical school, the foundation programme and vocational training. We sit our exams, receive our qualifications, and finally return with the glittering prize of our

DOI: 10.1201/9781003652045-36

professional membership to work within the world where our journey began. We treat our patients, who are usually grateful, and it all feels worthwhile. At times, however, we feel something different, as if an invisible barrier has sprung up between us and the people we care for. We see at those times that despite our best efforts, we aren't helping, and we see the fear and hurt in their eyes as they imagine that they are either beyond help, or that we have abandoned them. This is where the GP's journey diverges from that of the hero, for we have one final secret to learn.

Our training enables us to recognise the marks of disease in our patients' stories, to solve the diagnostic puzzle and prescribe an appropriate course of treatment, but in the process we have lost our sense of the stories themselves. Stories represent the thread that joins together our past, present and future into a coherent whole, a life that makes sense. Most people can accept pain, weakness and uncertainty better than we realise. What they cannot do without, however, is a way of coming to terms with their illness, of integrating a new and unsettling experience into their understanding of how the world works. This can lead to presentations that make little sense medically but are compelling in narrative terms: *"I haven't been drinking enough recently, and now my kidneys are hurting, so I need a scan because my dad had a tumour there."* We are in the realm of narrative here; the science is beside the point.

An effective narrative allows us to answer the questions raised by an illness: What has happened? Why? Why me? Why now? What might happen next and what can I do about it?[2] Just as we have a professional duty to reach some kind of diagnostic formulation, we also have a human one, to engage with our patients' perspective and agree a story that helps them make sense of their experience. The final stage of our journey, then, is a lesson learned not from our teachers, but from our patients: to continue to see their illness through the lens of medicine, but to see it also through that of narrative; to become heroes with bifocals.

References

1. Campbell Joseph, *The Hero with a Thousand Faces*. Pantheon Books, New York, 1949.

2. Helman CG. Diseases versus Illness in General Practice. *JRCGP*, 1981;31:548–552.

Flag-Waving and Learning to Dance*

Do you ever feel swamped during consultations? There can be a lot to keep track of: the patient's clinical problem, along with the "couple of other things while I'm here, doctor;" their ideas, concerns and expectations; the vaguely-remembered back-story in the notes; Quality and Outcomes Framework alerts; and an awareness of how late you're running and how long it is since you had anything to eat.

Red Flags always come first, indicators of potentially serious disease which cannot be ignored. The sight of a non-blanching rash in a hot child, or cachexia in the patient not seen for a while, triggers a familiar set of responses: focussed attention, the need for immediate and concrete action, and a knotted feeling in the stomach. There are Yellow Flags too, psycho-social predictors of prolonged illness, originally described in relation to new presentations of low back pain, but also applicable more generally. They include comorbid mental health problems, dissatisfaction with work, negative coping strategies and various fixed beliefs that can complicate recovery.[1] The response to recognising a Yellow Flag is less dramatic, an inward raising of the eyebrow rather than any immediate action.

The flag that no one wants to see is the heart-sink's Jolly Roger, flutter-ing menacingly in the breeze as the patient settles into their chair. Doctors sometimes experience strongly negative reactions – a sinking of the heart – on being consulted by particular patients, or types of patient, and it may be surmised that patients at times feel the same way about doctors.

---

* An earlier version of this piece was published as: Hoban B. Flag-waving and learning to dance. *Br J Gen Pract.* 2023 Feb 23;73(728):133. doi: 10.3399/bjgp23X732237. PMID: 36823053; PMCID: PMC9976818.

DOI: 10.1201/9781003652045-37

The reasons for such a response may not always be clear at the time, but it can have a profound impact on the course of a consultation.[2]

Flags are simply bits of information, cues indicating that the consultation may be headed in one direction or another if we allow it. There must be an almost infinite number of these, from a moistening of the eyes to a tone of voice or the repetition of certain words. Do we respond to all of them and risk losing our way in the conversation? How can we keep our focus in the right place with so much going on? There are times when the only flag I want to see is the chequered one signalling the end of the race.

Feeling our attention jump constantly from one cue to another is stressful, and the natural response is to resist, take control, square our shoulders and push through. This can work, in the sense of getting to the point where the consultation ends, although, depending on how assertive our patient is, it may actually make things more difficult and take longer, as well as reinforcing negative feelings on both sides.

I wonder if part of the difficulty stems from conflating focus and awareness, such that we keep too many things at the centre of our attention to be able to see any of them clearly, while neglecting what is at the edge. You may be familiar with a mindfulness exercise which involves staring at one spot on a wall while gradually extending the area around it of which we are aware: the point is that focus and awareness are complementary rather than exclusive. Perceived threats automatically trigger a narrowing of our perception, sharpening our focus at the expense of our peripheral vision, and this is a part of our involuntary response not just to Red Flags, but to anything that seems important. Like so many of our adaptive responses, however, it is non-specific and can easily become maladaptive, such that when the consultation requires subtlety and a light touch, these things move out of reach.

If there is an application to all of this, it is perhaps that we can keep track of more in our encounters with patients by not worrying about keeping track of quite so much, but instead agreeing with them what to focus on. The outcome of most consultations is not pre-determined, such that we can get there simply by facing the right way and moving forwards, wrestling our patients over the finish line. Rather, if we keep our attention on the person opposite us while maintaining an awareness of the surrounding landscape, we may go round in circles for a while, but are likely to arrive at a point we're both happy with sooner and with less expenditure of effort. After all, we wrestle opponents, but dance with partners.

References

1. Early identification and management of psychological risk factors ("yellow flags") in patients with low back pain: a reappraisal, Nicholas MK, Linton SJ, Watson PJ, Main CJ; "Decade of the Flags" Working Group, *Phys Ther* 2011;91(5):737–753. doi: 10.2522/ptj.20100224

2. Moscrop A. 'Heartsink' Patients in General Practice: A Defining Paper, Its Impact, and Psychodynamic Potential. *Br J Gen Pract* 2011;61(586):346–348. https://doi.org/10.3399/bjgp11X572490

Falling Off the Swing[*]

Life is full of periodicity: daily, weekly, monthly and annual patterns whose regularity generates a familiar rhythm. A certain amount of progression, perhaps, but mainly back and forth: wake and sleep, work and play, well and sick. In this sense, illness is something normal, to be borne while the pendulum swings that way in expectation that it will soon swing back again. Most of the time, it does, and it is easy for us to claim credit as doctors, even though we know that many problems get better by themselves. It's worth considering for a moment how this works, and what happens when it doesn't.

Acute infections, injuries and psychological traumas are not intrinsically self-limiting, but often seem to be because our natural response to them is so automatic and effective. Fever, pain, autonomic arousal, and distress are all components of this response, although it is easy to conflate them with the problem that triggered them. We do not experience disease directly, but only through the lens of illness, whose symptoms may indicate not that help is needed, but that it is already on the way.[1]

Labelling something as a symptom necessarily implies an underlying problem. Many "symptoms" in fact represent noise within the system, physiological processes that for some reason cross the threshold of our awareness, registering as a mismatch between how we feel and how we expect to feel.[2] This naturally gives rise to certain concerns, by addressing which we can resolve the mismatch, normalising it rather than looking for a cure. Even symptoms clearly related to long-term conditions naturally oscillate about a mean, and will at times peak for no reason. These are the times when patients

[*] An earlier version of this piece was published as: Hoban B. Falling off the swing. *Br J Gen Pract*. 2024 May 30;74(743):270. doi: 10.3399/bjgp24X738393. PMID: 38816250; PMCID: PMC11147466.

DOI: 10.1201/9781003652045-38

tend to seek help, but also when their symptoms are most likely to improve spontaneously, by a simple reversion to the mean.

Patients ride the oscillations of their health like a swing, waiting for things to get better one way or another, and holding on in confidence that this will indeed happen. The placebo effect describes the impact of this confidence on the degree and speed of their recovery, whether mediated by a pill, a person or some other element of their care.[3] Even simple observation is known to affect outcome measures: watching and waiting is not the same as just waiting.[4]

There are many whose recovery from illness is more complicated and at best partial, despite appropriate treatment and a lack of clear ongoing disease. It is as if the normal processes by which an illness resolves have shut down and the pendulum has become stuck at one extreme of its arc: adaptive responses become maladaptive; the statistical outlier pulls down the mean rather than reverting to it; symptoms multiply, and expectations become increasingly bleak. A quiet desperation starts to pervade the consultations, whose focus narrows in search of the elusive treatment, test or referral that will at last provide an answer.

Although doctor and patient both worry about missing a treatable underlying cause, there is by this time often no simple diagnosis that can make sense of it all. Whatever the original trigger, ongoing symptoms may instead be due to secondary factors such as deconditioning, autonomic dysfunction, altered processing of sensory signals, and loss of routine, purpose and social interaction.[5] Patients who have fallen off the swing of their daily lives find themselves unexpectedly on the floor, having lost momentum, sore and unsure of themselves. If they are to recover, they first need help to get off the ground, remount and restart those small regular movements that over time progress to a more graceful and effortless motion. Above all, they must have a reasonable expectation that these things are possible.

It is easy to feel as if we have nothing to offer patients suffering from chronic ill health, or even to resent them as a reminder of our failure to make things better. We cannot turn back the clock to a time before it all went wrong, but we can still entertain more modest aspirations. Healthy eating, a good night's sleep and a bit of fresh air will not fix anything, but small changes can still create conditions more favourable to some degree of meaningful recovery, and our role as doctors is to enable and support this, rather than to bring it about ourselves. Health too is dynamic, a daily succession of breaths in and out, systole and diastole, back and forth. We can draw our patients' attention to the small daily fluctuations in their symptoms that demonstrate this, help them to understand the physiological processes at work, and encourage a positive response that, over time, builds momentum. Most of all, though, we can just be there, a hand on the swing that gives someone the confidence to start moving again.

References

1. Helman C. Disease versus Illness in General Practice. *J R Coll Gen Pract* 1981;31:548–552.

2. Van den Bergh O, Witthöft M, Petersen S, Brown RJ. Symptoms and the Body: Taking the Inferential Leap. *Neurosci Biobehav Rev* 2017;74:185–203.

3. Enck P, Bingel U, Schedlowski M, Rief, W. The Placebo Response in Medicine: Minimize, Maximize or Personalize? *Nat Rev Drug Discov* 2013;12:191–204.

4. McCarney, R, Warner J, Iliffe S et al. The Hawthorne Effect: A Randomised, Controlled Trial. *BMC Med Res Methodol* 2007;7:30. https://doi.org/10.1186/1471-2288-7-30

5. Fink Per and Rosendal Marianne, eds., *Functional Disorders and Medically Unexplained Symptoms: Assessment and treatment.* Aarhus University Press, Aarhus, 2015.

Getting On with Strangers

A good doctor–patient relationship is one of the key features of successful general practice. I have received both compliments about how attentive and caring I was during one consultation, and complaints about how inattentive and uncaring I was during another, but little feedback about my clinical skills or adherence to national guidelines. Relationships matter, so how can we make sure that ours go well, and what does that look like? We first meet patients as strangers, but do we need to become friends? Are some doctors just better with people than others, or is getting on a skill that we can learn?

During a serious acute illness, the default relationship between a patient and their doctor has the clinical problem as the focus, the patient essentially passive, and the doctor taking charge. The dynamics of the situation are pretty straightforward. Most consultations are different, though: the problem is usually less clear-cut medically, and the patient's agenda determines the direction of travel more than the doctor's. The whole situation is more nuanced and uncertain, making it harder for either party to know how to relate to the other. The patient's position is: "I'll tell you why I'm here, but I need to know that you'll take me seriously,"[1] and the doctor's: "I'll do my best to help you, but I need to know that your expectations will be reasonable." Their relationship is defined by the way they bridge this gap, reaching out towards each other to make a connection. It is not an extra, or even a tool, but the operating system on which everything else runs.

There are times when this process doesn't go smoothly. The handshake perhaps meets a knuckle-bump or becomes a test of strength. Eric Berne famously encouraged us to seek adult–adult interactions, although we all sometimes find ourselves falling, or being pushed, into the role of parent or

DOI: 10.1201/9781003652045-39

child.[2] Emily and Laurence Alison's model illustrates this relational asymmetry by having a lion communicate with a mouse.[3] This can be a real challenge, and yet most patients and their doctors find a way to make it work: the secure child gently shows the coercive parent that cooperation works better than force; the strong lion gives the timid mouse courage to speak up. Some never do, but avoid each other when they can and dread the occasions on which they can't. The heart-sink is a relationship rather than a person.

Medical relationships, like others, can have a dark side too. When a complex patient with many needs and a difficult back-story at last finds a doctor able to understand and work with them, both may feel personally validated, even flattered, to have made such a special connection. There is also a risk of professional co-dependence, however, in which neither can ever challenge the other. Similarly, pairings based on transference and counter-transference can look successful, but actually reinforce each side's less healthy characteristics.[4] An authority figure and a pushover, or a victim and a saviour, may seek each other out simply because both parties know how the relationship works.

From a global and historical perspective, the way two people relate to each other has mainly depended on whether they were part of the same ethnic, kin or social group. *Impersonal prosociality*, the principle that one should instead extend the same courtesies to strangers as to friends, is, however, one of the hallmarks of modern Western culture, and linked with our idea of universal norms and the rule of law.[5] Although we're often wary of making eye contact with people we don't know, let alone talking to them, it can be surprisingly easy and rewarding, demonstrating that someone younger, better-dressed, or otherwise different in some way is still just a person like us. We are culturally wired to relate positively to each other, even to strangers, and we feel better when we do it.[6]

Our relationships with patients are more than just transactional, but they do not need to be based on affection or, necessarily, on duration. A good doctor–patient relationship is simply one that enables both parties to bridge the gap between them, and it is built jointly, whether in ten minutes or over twenty years. Doing this is a skill that can be learned and practised, but it starts with the recognition that, despite our differences, people are all made of the same stuff and are capable of working together, without our having to be anyone's friend or parent or rescuer. As demand for appointments grows, contact often remains remote, and personal continuity falls, my own patients often feel like strangers these days. Good to know, then, that strangers can still get on well together!

References

1. Croker J, Swancutt D, Roberts M, Abel G, Roland M, Campbell J. Factors Affecting Patients' Trust and Confidence in GPs: Evidence from the English National GP Patient Survey. *BMJ Open* 2013;3:e002762. https://doi.org/10.1136/bmjopen-2013-002762

2. Berne Eric, *Games People Play: the Psychology of Human Relationships*. Grove Press, New York, 1964.

3. Alison Emily, Alison Laurence, *Rapport: The Four Ways to Read People*. Vermilion, London, 2020.

4. Goldberg P. The Physician–Patient Relationship: Three Psychodynamic Concepts That Can Be Applied to Primary Care. *Arch Fam Med* 2000;9:1164–1168.

5. Henrich Joseph, *The WEIRDest People in the World: How the West Became Psychologically Peculiar and Particularly Prosperous*. Penguin, New York, 2021.

6. Keohane Joe, *The Power of Strangers: The Benefits of Connecting in a Suspicious World*. Penguin, New York, 2021.

Kobayashi Maru[*]

There is a kind of inevitability about the use of fighting metaphors in medicine, from the War on Cancer to treating people aggressively and battling an illness. If we are indeed at war with ill health then it is a conflict which, on the whole, we are used to winning. Even when we cannot cure or prevent it, we still expect to assert our control over disease by prolonging life as long as possible; and even at its very end, we do the same through the ritual of Treatment Escalation Plans, syringe drivers and End of Life pathways.

We are trained to do this, and it is difficult to stop and admit that at times our enemy has the upper hand. Even in cases where there is no immediate risk of death, but where chronic pain or other disabling symptoms drain the juice out of life, it feels wrong to tell patients that we have been outmanoeuvred and have nothing left to offer, and so we shrug our shoulders and add another prescription to the list. Maybe it will help.

A number of storylines within the *Star Trek* franchise refer to a combat simulation in which a stranded civilian starship, the *Kobayashi Maru*, must be rescued from hostile space, but in which any attempt to do so inevitably results in failure. The mission is impossible: it is intended as a test of character rather than tactical ability, of the capacity to recognise defeat when it is inevitable and act with equanimity. Captain Kirk refuses to accept this, however, and instead wins the unwinnable scenario by reprogramming the simulation. His behaviour is that of the archetypal hero, who must always overcome the monster or die trying. We can admire honourable defeat, but, given the choice, we prefer success. Acceptance is for losers, it would seem.

[*] An earlier version of this piece was published as: Hoban B. *Kobayashi Maru. Br J Gen Pract.* 2023 Oct 26;73(736):507. doi: 10.3399/bjgp23X735405. PMID: 37884377; PMCID: PMC10617972.

DOI: 10.1201/9781003652045-40

A similar emphasis on success and the nagging fear of failure pervade many consultations. Good doctors make things better, and we want to be good doctors, but what do we tell our patient when it becomes clear that whatever we do, we cannot win this fight? There is always room to bluff, to add more medication or make another referral, and yet, even as we do this, we know that we will have the same consultation again soon, and the bluff will have become less convincing. If all we have to offer is false hope and the illusion of control, perhaps it would be better for everyone if we admitted it.

I wonder if sometimes the difficulty we face as doctors is precisely that we try so hard, often heroically, to make things better, to fix the problem or manage the symptoms, when what many patients want above all is for us to acknowledge that, like them, we are helpless, that they face something truly unfixable and unmanageable, and that their experience of fighting an unwinnable battle makes complete sense. They already know they are beaten, and every well-intentioned suggestion is an implicit rebuke that they have given up too soon. They are demonstrating character by accepting what they must, and we are teasing them with promises of success.

The impact of recognising this can be transformative, changing the terms of the consultation from one in which the only possible outcomes are victory or failure to one in which doctor and patient become united against an infinitely powerful enemy. There is no shame in defeat here. Rather, in the face of such an opponent, success is measured in simple tasks achieved, in negotiating each day with its attendant challenges, in keeping going when keeping going seems impossible.

The danger of letting the moment pass, of holding onto our heroic aspirations, is that we start to see our patients as somehow at fault, ill because they have not tried hard enough to become well, and that we grow to resent them too for reminding us of our own inability to heal them. How many heart-sinks arise through just this process?

In our ongoing professional struggle on behalf of our patients, there will always be some battles that we can win and others that we cannot. By acknowledging this and allowing more than one kind of success, we may find ourselves redefining the terms of some of our most difficult consultations to make them winnable after all. Perhaps we are more like Captain Kirk than we realise.

Hyper-Burgers, Hyper-Medicine, and Making Sense of It All

Anyone seeking proof that life doesn't always live up to expectations need only consider the humble hamburger. Several fast-food chains have faced legal action over their alleged misrepresentation of meals, with claims that their burgers are smaller and less impressive than the picture on the menu.[1] Food photographers and stylists work hard to make their subjects look good, sometimes at the expense of accuracy. The issue is not necessarily one of honesty, though, but rather how something complex can be represented through a limited medium. Eating a burger will always be different to looking at it, so for an image to prepare us adequately for our meal, it has to convey visually something which is more than visual. In order to evoke something satisfying, rich, and bursting with filling, it must show something bigger and shinier, with more of its insides exposed, than the real thing. We could say that the image symbolises the experience of eating the burger rather than showing us perfectly what it looks like.

Hyperreality describes this tendency for symbols to come adrift from what they represent, and for the distinction between the two to be lost, so that it becomes unclear which is real, and what we should expect from our dinner.[2] We can see something similar in the way we think of medicine.

If you want to know what images we associate with healthcare, you can just google it: the typical picture is of a group of people in scrubs looking dynamic while interacting with some kind of cutting-edge tech; there is sometimes a supine patient in the background. What you absolutely don't see is two normally clothed people sitting together in a GP's consulting room trying to make sense of it all. We default to thinking of hospitals because they exemplify better the aspects of medicine which are specific to it, the technical as opposed to the relational, and the victory of science over disease.

DOI: 10.1201/9781003652045-41

Medicine has traditionally concerned itself with the diagnosis and treatment of disease, and there is a widespread view among patients, and some doctors, that this should still be our focus. According to this view, we live in a world of cause and effect, most people are healthy, and feeling ill means that you either have something proper wrong with you, or you're neurotic or pretending. Medicine has changed, however, and as a profession, we often concern ourselves more with things that are *disease-adjacent* such as risk, function and narrative. We regularly discuss with our patients the chance of developing cardiovascular disease over the coming decade in relation to primary prevention, or the likelihood that a given symptom is due to cancer, even though it usually isn't. We spend much of our time managing long-term conditions, which increasingly include functional problems such as fibromyalgia and various physical and psychological states that are certainly real, but have more to do with a harmful environment than disease. We treat where we can, but more often we support patients and help them find meaning in the chaos of their symptoms.[3] This is our hamburger.

There is a mismatch, then, between the concreteness of our healthcare symbols and the fuzziness of the reality they represent, and it is easy for experience to fall short of expectations. We have all looked after patients caught in the revolving door of repeated hospital admissions or specialist referrals, arranged with the honest intention of finally sorting things out, but leading instead to bitter disappointment at the point of discharge when once again, little has changed; medicine has failed to deliver. Maybe next time.

And yet, just as the hyper-burger symbolises something real, there is a deeper truth here towards which our symbols point. Most patients accept the limits of medicine and recognise that we are not miracle-workers. They do expect, however, that they will be heard, that their story will be believed, and that on some level it will make sense. You cannot eat a hyper-burger, and most of what patients need is not to be found in hospitals.[4] The images of hyper-medicine, of body scanners and experts, illustrate instead the universal need to be taken seriously and understood, whatever form that takes, and that should always be something we can deliver.

References

1. Burger King sued over Whopper burger, The Independent 4.9.23. https://www.independent.co.uk/news/uk/home-news/burger-king-whopper-lawsuit-b2403153.html

2. Baudrillard Jean, *Simulacra and Simulation*, originally published in French by Editions Galilée, 1981.

3. Frank Arthur, *The Wounded Storyteller: Body, Illness and Ethics*, 2nd Ed. University of Chicago Press, Chicago, 2013.

4. Shocking Food Photography Tricks You Should Know. https://fixthephoto.com/food-photography-tricks.html

Sick Notes and Culture*

It's difficult to know what to make of Prime Minister Rishi Sunak's comments about "sick-note culture" (Although the UK Prime Minister and government have changed since this piece was originally published, the issues raised by Rishi Sunak remain unresolved).[1] On the face of it, there is nothing unreasonable about reviewing the current system of sick certification by GPs, which can be a helpful part of patient care, but often represents just one more administrative burden in an already busy day. Even the fact that such a review is driven by financial pressures need not be a bad thing: the more people who are able to return to work and pay their taxes, the more money there is to pay out in benefits to those who depend on them. What stands out, however, is the reference to culture, implying not just that the system needs to be changed, but that it is somehow being subverted by a set of questionable values and norms. It is, in fact, well established that ideas and behaviours related to our health are universally influenced by cultural factors.[2] I would like to suggest three such factors that may be relevant to the observed increase in sick certification.

First, we have experienced a definite change in our attitude to ill health as a society, from carrying on regardless – now referred to as presenteeism – to stewarding our health as a precious resource. Since the COVID-19 pandemic, we think more readily of looking after others by isolating ourselves when ill, and looking after the health service by not risking illness at all. Even well before this, we were promoting vigilance for signs of meningitis, strokes, sepsis and cancer in terms reminiscent of terrorism awareness campaigns. Unattended luggage? *See it, say it, sorted!* Changes in a mole? *Get*

* An earlier version of this piece was published as: Hoban B. Sick notes and culture. *Br J Gen Pract*. 2024 Jun 27;74(744):315. doi: 10.3399/bjgp24X738633. PMID: 38936863; PMCID: PMC11221708.

DOI: 10.1201/9781003652045-42

it checked! Corresponding efforts to raise the profile of psychological problems are especially relevant, given the disproportionate rise in sick certification for mental ill health in young adults.[3, 4] We have encouraged people for years to be more open to the possibility of illness, and are now left with the unintended consequence that they have taken the message to heart.

Secondly, our focus in relation to ill health has shifted from acute problems to long-term physical and psychological conditions, some of which would once either have been considered normal, or swept under the carpet.[5] Arthur Frank identifies three main narratives in relation to illness: Restitution, or simply getting better; Quest, or personal growth through adversity; and Chaos, in which things don't make sense, they simply happen as they will.[6] Any ongoing condition necessarily excludes the first, and any attempt to make sense of it naturally avoids the last. The only positive story left to the chronically unwell, then, is to accept what they must and look for some good in it. To tell someone in this position that they are either not sick enough to qualify for benefits, or not trying hard enough to get better, rather misses the point. It also raises the question of how we decide who can occupy the sick role, which brings us to our third cultural change.

Talcott Parsons originally described the sick role as one of several ways in which society recognises deviance from accepted norms of behaviour, other examples including criminality and insanity.[7] According to this view, if you can't fit in, there must be something wrong with you. Our current ideas of normality are more descriptive than prescriptive, and we view diversity as something positive rather than an anomaly needing to be legitimised. As a result, we have come to see ourselves as defined less by the things we have in common, and more by the things that make us distinctive. In this context, poor health easily becomes one of the facets of a person's identity, and attempts to challenge this are likely to come over as personally invalidating.

The difficulty with this position is that it obliges the system to pay benefits to someone purely on the basis of how they see themselves. As doctors, we try to take what patients tell us at face value and be supportive where we can; we have to choose our battles carefully, and we have no way, ultimately, of verifying someone's story. Mr Sunak may therefore be right that we are not the best people to question someone's reported inability to work. The idea that this can be done fairly and objectively by someone else, however, seems dubious. In order to be fit for work, a person must be capable of more than simply carrying out in isolation the tasks required by their role: they must be able to do so repeatedly, to a consistent standard, and in a way that represents a reasonable balance of benefits and burdens to them. If working in toxic conditions for a pittance leaves you too exhausted or stressed to do anything else, you are not fit to work by any reasonable standard, or by any standard at all for long, even if you can turn a handle or click a mouse when asked.

Where does this leave us? The idea that we can consider ill health without taking into account our wider cultural context is a non-starter. We might rather consider to what extent we have contributed to the current culture by setting out to change the way people relate to their health, and to healthcare: in lighting a candle of increased illness awareness, we have also cast a shadow of increased illness behaviour. There are unlikely to be any simple solutions, but a new sick-certification service will need to demonstrate that it can cut costs without being punitive and arbitrary, or increasing demand for appointments as patients seek help in appealing decisions made against them.

References

1. Press release: PM to overhaul benefits system and tackle Britain's "sick note culture" in welfare reform speech. http://gov.uk/government/news/pm-to-overhaul-benefits-system-and-tackle-britains-sick-note-culture-in-welfare-reform-speech

2. Helman Cecil, *Culture, Health and Illness*, 5th ed., CRC Press, Boca Raton, FL, 2007.

3. Simon AS. Wessely: "Every Time We Have a Mental Health Awareness Week My Spirits Sink" *BMJ* 2017;358:j4305. https://doi.org/10.1136/bmj.j4305

4. No health without mental health: a cross-governmental mental health outcomes strategy for people of all ages, HM Government, 2011. https://assets.publishing.service.gov.uk/media/5a7c348ae5274a25a914129d/dh_124058.pdf

5. What we know about the UK's working-age health challenge, The Heath Foundation, 2023.https://www.health.org.uk/publications/long-reads/what-we-know-about-the-uk-s-working-age-health-challenge

6. Frank Arthur, *The Wounded Storyteller: Body, Illness and Ethics*. University of Chicago Press, Chicago, 1997.

7. Parsons Talcott, *The Social System*. Free Press, Glencoe, IL, 1951.

Seeing and Hearing*

Ask any doctor, and they'll tell you that talking to patients can be difficult. Mind you, ask any patient and they'll tell you that talking to doctors can be really difficult too. The Consultation, that every-day and much-discussed occasion during which both processes occur, can sometimes feel like a shared illusion of communication, which leaves both parties none the wiser.[1]

Doctors are routinely trained in communication skills now, although there are times when what I really want to do is to send my patients on the course. Even as I listen, I find myself willing the person opposite to give me just a little more to work with, or a little less. There are so many potential barriers to understanding each other, from the lack of a shared language, verbal or non-verbal, to a divergence of expectations or simple time pressure. And yet, I have a suspicion that what underlies our difficulties is often something else.

Patients sometimes talk in ways that make little sense to us, repeating seemingly unimportant details, abruptly changing subject and even contradicting themselves. We sit patiently, waiting for "usable intel," or grab hold of the first thing we can. Even when a coherent thread emerges and we offer a diagnosis and management plan, the response can be surprisingly cool. What escapes us is that people talk like this for the same reason they extend their hand on first meeting someone: not to invite scrutiny, but to bridge a gap.

In general, people overestimate the extent to which this is necessary.[2] We worry that strangers are different and won't understand or like us, and this can make it difficult to talk about things that matter, especially with

* An earlier version of this piece was published as: Hoban B. Seeing and hearing. *Br J Gen Pract.* 2023 Mar 30;73(729):172. doi: 10.3399/bjgp23X732429. PMID: 36997223; PMCID: PMC10049618.

DOI: 10.1201/9781003652045-43

someone as famously busy as a doctor. Judging by their comments, patients regularly worry that they're wasting our time or that we'll think they are, and much of what they say is intended simply to engage our attention and sympathy. We tend to question our competence and fret about missing a diagnosis, but the person in the other chair is usually more concerned to know whether we're listening and taking them seriously.[3]

Connecting is the first of Neighbour's five checkpoints in the consultation, not just a verbal or literal handshake, but rather something that must be maintained in order for effective communication to take place.[4] This is what is meant by *rapport*, a state of mutual responsiveness to which both parties contribute, but which in a medical context is primarily the doctor's responsibility.[5]

Curiously, the research literature on rapport seems largely based on data from police and counter-terrorism interviews, which has to represent a tougher crowd than any Monday morning surgery! Broadly speaking, techniques used to promote rapport fall into three categories: personalising an interaction; presenting an approachable demeanour; and paying attention.[6] In the consultation this covers the familiar ground of keeping an open posture, nodding, summarising, asking about patients' concerns and dragging our eyes away from the computer. It also includes asking questions that demonstrate interest in someone's circumstances, using their name and, in small doses, talking about yourself.

These are all things we can do without too much difficulty, and they may well improve our consultations: doctors do generally listen and try to help, but often give little indication of it, leaving patients to project their anxieties onto the blank screen of a resting face. At its heart, though, rapport is about attitude rather than skill. It means acknowledging a patient, not just as a puzzle for us to solve or an obstacle to negotiate before we can go home, but as someone like us with reasonable concerns and a valid claim on our attention.[7] In this sense, it depends less on particular "moves" than on values like honesty, empathy, autonomy and respect.[8]

Being able to talk well with patients, especially those with whom we don't naturally get on, is an ability at once mundane and elusive, but it is important, the hallmark of the "virtuoso GP."[9] And, like so many other important things, it boils down to a simple principle: seeing and hearing someone as another person and letting them know that they've been seen and heard.

References

1. "The great enemy of communication, we find, is the illusion of it." Variously quoted and attributed but originally from an article entitled "Is Anybody Listening?" by William H. Whyte published in *Fortune* magazine, September 1950.

2. Keohane Joe, *The Power of Strangers: The Benefits of Connecting in A Suspicious World*. Penguin, New York, 2022.

3. Howard S. GPs caught in media menopause spotlight. *BMJ* 2022;379:o2841. https://doi.org/10.1136/bmj.o2841

4. Neighbour Roger, *The Inner Consultation: How to Develop an Effective and Intuitive Consulting Style*. 1st edition. Springer, Cham, 1987.

5. Moulton Liz, *The Naked Consultation: A Practical Guide to Primary Care Consultation Skills*. Radcliffe, London, 2007.

6. Gabbert F, Hope L, Luther K, Wright G, Ng M, Oxburgh G. Exploring the Use of Rapport in Professional Information-Gathering Contexts by Systematically Mapping the Evidence Base. *Appl Cognit Psychol*. 2021;35:329–341. https://doi.org/10.1002/acp.3762

7. Ballatt J, Campling P. *Intelligent Kindness: Reforming the Culture of Healthcare*. RCPsych Publications, 2011.

8. Alison Emily, Alison Laurence, *Rapport: The Four Ways to Read People*. Vermillion, London, 2020.

9. Senior T. Virtuoso General Practice. *Br J Gen Pract* 2022;72(721):395. https://doi.org/10.3399/bjgp22X720425

Scientists after All

It's difficult to imagine being a doctor without a solid grounding in the natural sciences, in terms of both a scientific way of thinking and all the more tangible benefits that science brings to medicine. And yet despite all that science has to tells us in general terms about people and how to care for them, it is often harder to pin down on specifics.

Consider a randomised controlled trial comparing a new treatment with an old one. If we measure a specified outcome like a 3-point reduction in symptom score by day 7, we can either express results in terms of probability (you are 10% more likely to be feeling better with the new treatment) or Number Needed to Treat (of ten patients, one will feel better). Even if the results are strongly positive, however, a meaningful benefit depends on measuring the right outcome, and a large net benefit across a group of patients may still conceal significant variation within the group and mean less for each individual. We tend to gloss over this and hide behind more concrete positions: this treatment works, that one doesn't.[1]

The science provides an evidence base for our practice, but only in terms that can be easily measured, and knowing how to apply this evidence to the patient sat in front of us can be a real challenge. It's also clear that patients aren't just passive vehicles of disease waiting for us to look under the bonnet and effect a technical fix: they have their own concerns and priorities, and may prefer having these addressed to being presented with a solution to a problem that exists more in their doctor's mind than their own.

It is clear, then, that we need something else as well as science: humanities, empathy, kindness, narrative, wisdom, communication skills; in any case, something that does the things that science cannot. This is the origin

DOI: 10.1201/9781003652045-44

of concepts like holistic practice, the doctor–patient relationship, and the management of uncertainty, which we tend to associate with the GP brand. When push comes to shove, though, we often revert to a more scientific approach focussed on finding and treating disease.

There is a point, then, where it becomes reasonable to ask whether science and our *something else* are really complementary opposites, like left and right hands working together, or simply values at odds with each other, like high fashion and comfortable shoes. If they balance each other, we can have as much as we like of one, as long as we have enough of the other; if they conflict, we may have to choose one at the other's expense. It may help to consider first what science is really about, and where it came from.

The scientific method has traditionally been about three things: empiricism, reductionism and generalisation. It has dealt only with what can be observed directly, breaking down complex wholes into simple parts, and identifying these components strictly in terms of their individual properties. Context and ambiguity have not been welcome.

The development of the scientific method in medieval Europe coincided with a shift away from the existing kin-based society, in which individuals functioned as nodes in a complex network of family ties, and in which identity and behavioural norms were determined by the context of interpersonal relationships. It was gradually replaced by one in which family ties became more limited, behavioural norms were based on rules rather than context, and individuals could define themselves through things like their marriage choices, occupation and place of residence. As society became less relational and more individual, people started to view the material world in similar terms.[2] Classical science takes as its starting point a universe made up of discrete things with defined properties, relating to each other by fixed laws.

Quantum physics, by contrast, looks not at the macroscopic world with which we are familiar, but at the subatomic world on which it is built, inhabited by particles and waves rather than physicists and apple trees. On this scale things are very different: quantum objects do not move smoothly like billiard balls from A to B, but appear here or there based on a probability distribution which may assign maximal values to points between A and B, but also includes non-zero probabilities for many others, including Alpha Centauri and your washing machine. Furthermore, it is no longer possible for us to assume the role of objective observers: we are necessarily a part of the system in view, and the act of making an observation changes the system. How then can we know anything? If every detail we consider contains an infinite world of possibilities, collapsed to a point by our observation, does that then mean that there exists an infinite number of worlds in which every possible outcome takes place? Perhaps the difficulty lies in talking about *changing* things: it assumes that an object is secretly one thing until we come along to apply our tape measure and it becomes something else. It is perhaps more accurate to say that we *define* things by measuring them, but not just in a narrow scientific sense: rather, in the sense that on the quantum scale any two objects are *undefined* until they touch, when their properties and behaviour arise from the way they *relate* to each other.[3] Fire a stream of electrons at a target and you'll see successive impacts suggesting that electrons are particles; interpose a diffraction grating and the resulting interference pattern will persuade you that they are waves. Characteristics do depend on context after all!

Macroscopic objects are simply large groupings of quantum objects, like populations of patients in a drug trial, in which all the variations and kinks balance each other out, giving the impression of homogeneity. The difference between classical and quantum science is one of scale: one describes the river, flowing always into the sea; the other, the individual ripples and eddy currents that make it up and flow in all sorts of directions.

I often feel a tension between my professional obligations to apply good science, and to care for patients as individuals. Which is it to be? I suppress a vague sense of guilt every time I ignore the Quality and Outcomes Framework pop-up in the corner of the screen to let the patient finish their story, and I realise that I won't shock anyone reading this by admitting it. But what if by focussing on the relational aspects of the consultation I get something medical wrong? What if I'm not *sciencey* enough? I find it comforting to know that the material world our science describes is at its heart contextual and relational, and that what seem at first like two opposing ideals are, in fact, the extremes on a scale of magnification. The question is not whether we apply science or choose instead one of the woollier alternatives with which we like to contrast it, but whether in a given case to zoom in or out to see the picture more clearly. The true facts often emerge only when we focus on the seemingly woolly; the real story arises not just through our skilled questioning, but through our active participation in it. General Practice is not science-lite, but cutting-edge, and we shouldn't be afraid to own it.

References

1. Quick summaries of evidence-based medicine provided by an independent panel of experts mainly working in the USA. https://thennt.com

2. Henrich Joseph, *The WEIRDest People in the World: How the West Became Psychologically Peculiar and Particularly Prosperous*. Penguin, London, 2021.

3. Rovelli Carlo, *Helgoland*. Allen Lane, London, 2021.

Retrospectoscopy

Doctor, I've just had this letter from the hospital.

Ah yes, your retrospectoscopy results: if only we'd had these before!

How is it that something can seem so obvious in hindsight, when at the time it was anything but? If we think of life as a chain of events stretching from the past into the future like a string of beads, then what we see clearly from a point of view in the future should be equally clear from our current viewpoint in the present, and to be caught out by events must be due to a simple failure to look ahead.

I may regret choosing one set of lottery numbers over another when the winners are drawn. It would be misleading, however, to say that I had picked the *wrong* numbers: in a fair game, the result simply cannot be determined in advance. It is therefore possible, at least in principle, for the view through the retrospectoscope to have a clarity which is both compelling and false.

The reason for this is that life is a good deal more complicated than a string of beads, and more like a web of interconnected nodes, from each of which we can pass to any number of others, such that there is a virtually infinite number of pathways through the web. At any given point, what happens next is influenced by more factors than we can account for. We can certainly make our string of beads, but only by deciding which nodes to connect and which to ignore: we choose our narrative, linking selected facts to explain how we came to be where we are, although we do so at the expense of the bigger picture.

DOI: 10.1201/9781003652045-45

This causal asymmetry is evident whenever we make decisions. We generally accept that things might not work out the way we think they will, but we proceed by taking as our starting point the outcome we're hoping for, while also considering a number of other possible scenarios: how likely they seem; what impact they might have; how we would feel about them; and what stories we would tell in hindsight to explain them. If you woke up on the Coronary Care Unit after a heart attack, would you blame yourself for not having taken a statin? Or would you feel cheated if you'd had a heart attack despite taking one?

We can apply the same process to our safety netting in the consultation by planning for things to go well, anticipating the ways in which they might also go wrong, and advising our patients accordingly, so that we are left with a reasonable narrative whatever happens. If we were right first time, it's a simple success story; if things take an unexpected turn for the worse but the patient knows what to do, the success in narrative terms is greater rather than less. If, on the other hand, we foresee that our actions might lead to an outcome which we could never justify in hindsight, we will know that we need to rethink our plan.

> *Now, Mrs Jones, everything looks fine, but I'd just like to do one more thing to make sure you're going to be okay.*
>
> *My goodness, doctor, what's that?!*
>
> *Don't worry, Mrs Jones, this is a modified retrospectoscope with a state-of-the-art anticipatory filter. It lets me see what things might look like in hindsight a few days from now.*
>
> *Are you sure? It looks awfully like something my children put together...*
>
> *Not at all. In the future, all doctors will have one. In fact, we'll wonder why we didn't realise sooner how useful they could be.*

Relational Care

It has become generally accepted that personally continuous care is good care, and the discussion is currently more concerned with whether or not it is achievable in a system universally acknowledged to be struggling. It is clear, however, that continuity arises more readily in some settings than others,[1] and that even where it flourishes, it still needs help to do so: practices with a high degree of personal continuity tend to have systems that actively promote it, both by enabling patients to see their own doctor, and by making it more difficult for them to see someone else. The fact that such systems should be necessary makes sense in the context of changes that have been taking place in UK general practice over a matter of decades.

Continuity of care was originally part of a package which also included a high proportion of single-handed practices, 24-hour responsibility for patients, freedom for doctors to apply a limited medical knowledge base as they thought best, and a standard of care set by their professional colleagues. This landscape, in which personal continuity arose naturally, has now changed: group practices providing in-hours care only, and including part-time salaried GPs and non-medical professionals, are now the norm, and care is standardised and judged against patients' expectations. The government has gained control over the system; doctors have gained the freedom to have a life outside the surgery; and patients have gained – at least in theory – unlimited access to textbook medicine, regardless of who provides it. In the light of all these changes, what sense does it make to pursue continuity of care in isolation from the other elements of practice that used to make it the norm?

DOI: 10.1201/9781003652045-46

Ask a patient which doctor they'd like to see, and the answer will tend to be: anyone; their usual doctor; a doctor suited to help with a particular problem; or a *different* doctor to the one they usually see. In practical terms, access is often valued more highly than continuity for acute problems, especially among less-affluent patients.[2, 3] What is it, then, that makes continuity of care so beneficial, and might there be ways of achieving the same benefits in a system that is becoming less continuous?[4]

Sidaway-Lee and colleagues consider a number of mechanisms through which continuity of care might improve outcomes, identifying knowledge, trust, and empathy as especially significant.[5] In the context of the consultation, knowledge implies more than a simple familiarity with the facts of the case, however thorough, but rather a degree and breadth of disclosure which a patient chooses to make to a doctor they trust, and to which the doctor responds empathetically. Similarly, trust goes beyond what can be assumed from the letters before and after someone's name: it suggests confidence based on a prior knowledge of their ability and character. Empathy is only possible where one person knows and trusts another sufficiently to identify with their experience. These are interactions that only take place within a successful partnership between two people. Relationships tend to be built over time, and yet a long relationship is not necessarily a happy one, or a short one necessarily superficial. A longstanding doctor–patient relationship can lead to collusion, blind spots and resentment, while a new one can bring a fresh perspective.

Perhaps there is something more subtle at stake. On a procedural level, care is arguably more continuous than ever before: a doctor in Liverpool should, in theory, have access to all the relevant information about a patient from Aberystwyth, treat them according to the same medical evidence base, and expect the same results.[6] Patients routinely assume that what happens in one part of the health service is immediately known throughout, as if it were an organic whole. I have often been mistaken by patients for colleagues with whom I share no distinguishing physical characteristics; we are sometimes seen not as ourselves, but as local avatars of The Doctor, generic portals through which users access the system. This suggests that the real issue is not so much the presence or absence of continuity, but whether we construe continuity in primarily organisational or relational terms, and which kind we value more.

It is worth considering, then, that personal continuity of care may not simply be an accidental victim of the changes taking place within the health service, but the unavoidable casualty of a paradigm shift from the tailored care of individuals to the systematic care of whole populations. We cannot turn back the clock, but we can be proactive in pursuing those elements of practice that foster good working relationships with patients, and which have been shown to be successful in the context of such relationships: listening; building rapport and goodwill; sharing uncertainty and decision-making; and fostering accountability. In our current direction of travel towards ever-larger practices, we may also need to consider the upper size limit that would still allow patients to get to know even a few clinicians, so as to be confident of seeing at least one familiar face when they need to; and which would allow those clinicians to collaborate effectively in caring for them. We must pursue what continuity is available to us, but we can still practice relational care with what we have.

References

1. Te Winkel MT, Slottje P, de Kruif AJ, Lissenberg-Witte BI, van Marum RJ, Schers HJ, Uijen AA, Bont J, Maarsingh OR. Otto General Practice and Patient Characteristics Associated with Personal Continuity: Mixed Methods Study. *BJGP* 2022. https://doi.org/10.3399/BJGP.2022.0038

2. Aboulghate A, Abel G, Elliott MN, Parker RA, Campbell J, Lyratzopoulos G, Roland M. Do English Patients Want Continuity of Care, and Do They Receive It? *BJGP* 2012;62(601):e567–e575. https://doi.org/10.3399/bjgp12X653624

3. Baker R, Boulton M, Windridge K, Tarrant C, Bankart J, Freeman GK. Interpersonal Continuity of Care: A Cross-sectional Survey of Primary Care Patients' Preferences and Their Experiences. *BJGP* 2007;57:283–290.

4. Tammes P, Morris RW, Murphy M, Salisbury C. Is Continuity of Primary Care Declining in England? Practice-level Longitudinal Study From 2012 to 2017. *Br J Gen Pract* 2021;71(707):e432–e440. https://doi.org/10.3399/BJGP.2020.0935

5. Sidaway-Lee K, Denis Pereira Gray OBE, Harding A, Evans P. What Mechanisms Could Link GP Relational Continuity to Patient Outcomes? *Br J Gen Pract* 2021;71(707):278–281. https://doi.org/10.3399/bjgp21X716093

6. Burch P, Whittaker W, Bower P, Checkland, K. Factors Affecting the Experience of Joined-up, Continuous Primary Care in the Absence of Relational Continuity: An Observational Study *Br J Gen Pract* 2024;74(742):e300–e306. https://doi.org/10.3399/BJGP.2023.0208

Uncertainty, Placebos, and Travelling with Confidence

As in life, few things in medicine are certain, and in any clinical encounter, we must consider carefully the chances that someone's symptoms have a serious underlying cause, that a given intervention will be effective, or that we have missed something important. Uncertainty can be reduced or mitigated, but it remains a fact of life, defining the terrain across which doctors and patients must make their way.[1] There are guidelines and expert opinions to help us, like maps on which the preferred route is clearly marked, but they are not always a good match for the landscape in which we find ourselves. The path between where we are now and where we need to be has a habit of petering out, and blood tests and scans do not always help, sometimes giving us just a more technical class of uncertainty. From a patient's perspective, too, the road leading from illness back to health can be difficult to follow, even when we have a reasonable working diagnosis and management plan.

In the absence of complete certainty, then, any course of action must involve a step into the unknown, requiring at least a basic confidence that we are not walking into disaster. Can any of us be totally sure that the world will still be here tomorrow morning? And yet we set our alarms all the same, just as patients take their medicine with the expectation that it will do them good. The placebo effect is the clearest demonstration that expectations matter, and it is about people as much as pills.[2, 3] Patients responding more strongly to placebos tend to score highly in personality tests for extraversion, agreeableness and openness to experience, as opposed to caution, rationality and reserve; and their doctors consult with attention, warmth, thoughtful silence and, perhaps most importantly, confidence.

As a profession, we are ambivalent about placebos. The designers of every Randomised Controlled Trial acknowledge their importance, although

DOI: 10.1201/9781003652045-47

their deliberate use seems too much like a confidence trick[4] for us to view them as legitimate clinical tools.[5] A con is a predatory act of manipulation achieved by deceit, but the surprising truth about placebos is that they can still help even if everyone knows exactly what they are.[6] A patient's confidence may be focussed on a particular treatment, and originate in a positive interaction with their doctor, but it is still their confidence that produces the observed therapeutic effect. The miracle cure and the charismatic super-doctor are context-specific examples of this which we might hesitate to endorse, but there is no reason why the same effect might not simply enable someone to feel better following their consultation, without the need for either.

Plenty of people visit their doctor because they want to be told what's wrong and given a prescription. Many also come in order to share their uncertainties, and together find a reasonable way through them. Our role is not to pretend that we have all the answers, but nor is it to sit on the sidelines simply because we don't. If we are to empower patients by giving them the confidence to step into the unknown, we cannot do it primarily by being certain, but by acting in good faith when there is no certainty, just as bravery does not mean being fearless, but rather taking action in the face of our fears. Our base may be located within the citadel of medical knowledge, but I would like to suggest that we come into our own as GPs when we agree to accompany the sick on their journey outside its walls, out of neither ignorance nor recklessness, but in order that they should not have to travel there alone. We have a professional obligation to keep up to date, and our patients will hopefully take it as read that we know what we are doing. They are more likely to thank us, though, for also having taken the trouble to walk alongside them when they needed it. The drug "doctor," like any other, may function at times as a placebo,[7] but it is nevertheless an effective means of helping those forced to cross the rough ground of illness, and one which they still seem to appreciate.

References

1. Han Paul KJ, *Uncertainty in Medicine: A Framework for Tolerance.* Oxford University Press, Oxford, 2021.

2. Finniss DG, Kaptchuk TJ, Miller F, Benedetti F. Biological, Clinical and Ethical Advances of Placebo Effects. *Lancet* 2010;375:686–695.

3. Enck P, Bingel U, Schedlowski M, & Rief W. The Placebo Response in Medicine: Minimize, Maximize or Personalize? *Nat Rev Drug Discov* 2013;12:191–204.

4. Konnikova Maria, *The Confidence Game: The Psychology of the Con and Why We Fall For It Every Time.* Canongate Books, Edinburgh, 2016.

5. Fässler M, Gnädinger M, Rosemann T, Biller-Andorno N. Placebo Interventions in Practice: A Questionnaire Survey on the Attitudes of Patients and Physicians. *Br J Gen Pract* 2011;61(583):101–107. https://doi.org/10.3399/bjgp11X556209

6. von Wernsdorff M, Loef M, Tuschen-Caffier B, Schmidt S. Effects of Open-label Placebos in Clinical Trials: A Systematic Review and Meta-analysis. *Sci Rep.* 2021 Feb 16;11(1):3855. https://doi.org/10.1038/s41598-021-83148-6. Erratum in: *Sci Rep.* 2021 Aug 25;11(1):17436. PMID: 33594150; PMCID: PMC7887232.

7. Bar-Haim S. 'The Drug Doctor': Michael Balint and the Revival of General Practice in Postwar Britain. *Hist Workshop J* Autumn 2018;86:114–132. https://doi.org/10.1093/hwj/dby017

Medically Explained Symptoms

Symptoms are the raw material upon which doctors exercise their craft, the base metal our patients carry to surgery in bulging sacks and on rusty wheelbarrows to be transmuted into diagnostic gold. Or perhaps they are more like precious objects concealed in the lining of a jacket, reluctantly displayed when necessity demands, and we are the pawnbroker, appraising the value of Aunt Agatha's pearls and issuing cash against them. *Yes, I see what you mean, backache radiating to the leg, unpleasant but nothing unusual. A slipped disc: keep it moving and take the pills and it should be fine.* There are certainly a weighing and an exchange that take place between doctor and patient: symptoms for diagnosis; a mystery for an explanation; a crisis for a way forward. This is the fundamental transaction of the consultation.

The idea that someone's symptoms might not have an explanation is therefore highly disturbing, and the label of Medically Unexplained Symptoms is less of a diagnosis, adding nothing beyond a shrug of the medical shoulders, and more of a signal that no further efforts towards diagnosis will be made. The pearls are fake: it's time to go now, and please don't make a fuss.

Maybe the key to making sense of this is to consider more closely what we mean when we talk about symptoms in the first place. Strictly speaking, the term assumes that a particular sensation or occurrence is *symptomatic* of an underlying disease, when in fact complaints like headaches, indigestion and tiredness are so prevalent as to be essentially normal.[1] Similarly, we often view such things as fever, pain, vasodilation or tachycardia as unnatural, signs that something has gone wrong inside us and that our body is under attack. In reality, they are all things our body does itself, indicators of our response to some trigger or disease against which we are already

DOI: 10.1201/9781003652045-48

defending ourselves. This may seem like splitting hairs, but the corollary is that our body may at times also behave in a similar way in the absence of disease. How then can we tell whether someone's presentation has a significant underlying cause or not? The honest answer is of course that we often can't, but that we can still take whatever action seems appropriate. In deciding how we go about this, a combination of the patient's level of concern, the doctor's global impression, and the overall clinical context may, in any case, be a better guide than lists of symptoms, many of which are commonplace and non-specific. We treat, reassure, observe or investigate as the situation demands.

In the end, symptoms may remain unexplained despite our best efforts, and much of what our patients bring us can never be transformed into gold or pawned, no matter how hard we try. Attempts to extract diagnostic currency may not just be futile, but ultimately miss the point: the value of Aunt Agatha's pearls may be entirely sentimental, but they are still valuable. Likewise, what people confide in their doctor may not always tell us much about what is wrong with them, but it will say something about their circumstances, their priorities and their concerns. Medically Explained Symptoms have their place, of course, but let's not make the mistake of assuming that a strictly medical understanding of what our patients tell us is either the only kind, or necessarily the best. Indeed, there may be times when the most valuable outcome of a consultation is a more effective partnership between doctor and patient as they come to understand each other and learn to work together. There is now a solid evidence base demonstrating that personal continuity of care in General Practice, which enables such collaboration, is associated with measurably better clinical outcomes, including reduced mortality.[2] It may therefore be that the best way to spot the symptoms of serious disease is not always to be looking for them. If we accept instead the sentimental value of imitation pearls and get to know them well, we may more easily recognise the real thing when it comes along.

References

1. McAteer A, Elliott A, Hannaford P. Ascertaining the Size of the Symptom Iceberg in a UK-wide Community-based Survey. *BJGP* 2011. https://doi.org/10.3399/bjgp11X548910

2. Pereira-Grey D, Sidaway-Lee K, White E, Thorne A, Evans P. Improving Continuity: THE Clinical Challenge. *InnovAiT*, 1–11. https://doi.org/10.1177/1755738016654504

Eating the Elephant or Riding It

Nobody goes to the doctor's just because there's something wrong with them, but because whatever is wrong has crossed some threshold of personal significance in terms of either its effect on their life or what it might otherwise mean to them: a cough shouldn't last this long; I can't afford to be off sick; my dad had this, and he died. It is this significance, which is by definition individual, that drives the consultation and must be addressed alongside the usual business of diagnosis and treatment, the patient's agenda as well as the doctor's. It can be difficult to ask someone what they think is going on, what they're worried will happen as a result, or what help they're looking for without provoking that familiar verbal slap on the wrist, *I Don't Know, You're The Doctor*. A lot of people find it a challenge to answer these questions, perhaps worrying that they'll look foolish, or that mentioning something truly awful will make it more real. Some patients offer a respectable set of concerns with which to test the waters, only making a fuller disclosure if they're sure of a fair hearing.

The reason this matters is that the point of the consultation is primarily to deal with the patient's agenda, not the doctor's. Most patients are happy to leave the technical aspects of their care to the expert, but they still want to feel involved in making decisions and have confidence that the outcome will meet their needs as they see them.[1] If the process is too one-sided, it is easy for us to act in a way which represents good medical practice, but completely fails to address these needs. There are many patients around whom considerable medical activity takes place, who still complain that no-one's doing anything to help them: this may not technically be accurate, but it is true in the sense that no-one has yet offered them what they were

DOI: 10.1201/9781003652045-49

looking for, or explained why they can't, which amounts to the same thing from their point of view.

Our normal practice in any consultation is to address either the substance, the impact, or the meaning of the patient's presentation: we treat, mitigate or explain as the situation requires. Each of these approaches is similar in that it aims to make the problem smaller, more manageable. And yet, there is sometimes a sense of something missed, or skirted around, an elephant in the room whose trunk, ears, legs and tail we take note of without ever putting them together. What may be needed at such times, and what our patients may want most, is for us to assemble this elephant, to make the problem larger rather than smaller. When dealing with one complaint merely leads to the next, when every answer prompts a *Yes, but...* and when our heart sinks at the prospect of another frustrating consultation, it may be time to look for a bigger picture.

Pointing out that someone seems to have a lot of medical problems, reflecting on the difficulties this must cause them, and asking if they've ever wondered whether there might be a reason for it all can feel risky. A patient may not be in a position to look beyond their immediate concerns, and there is a danger of implying that they are taking up too much of our time, or worse, that it's all in their head. Perhaps the biggest risk is that the answer to our question will be hard for us to hear, an elephant that we cannot control. Discussing rare diseases,[2] adverse childhood experiences,[3] neurodivergence,[4] or contested medical disorders[5] can take us beyond our zones of both comfort and competence, a form of cross-cultural encounter that pulls out from under our feet the rug of familiar context, safe assumptions and shared language. In fact, this is often how patients feel when they consult a doctor![6] In these situations, it is easy to fall into power struggles about whose way of seeing things we should adopt, when there may be a way of accommodating both our perspectives.[7]

Patients who have already worked out that there is something else underlying their symptoms will not feel better if we try to shrink the world of their experience with bland reassurances or by trying a bit of this or that medication. Establishing a bigger picture may not fix anything, but it can help patients to make sense of what is happening and come to an understanding with their doctor about how to approach the more day-to-day issues that arise within the context of this larger view. If all we have to offer are platitudes and cures, we will be stuck forever trying to eat the elephant in the room – a possibility in theory, but rarely in practice. If instead we can understand and engage with our patients' point of view, we may be in a position to do far more: validate, support, enable and occasionally say sorry when we get it wrong. When we find ourselves getting bogged down in consultations, it may be time to ask those risky questions and start putting together the parts in front of us, remembering that elephants are also powerful beasts of burden, able to carry heavy loads and passengers on their journey through difficult terrain in safety.

References

1. Protheroe J, Bower P. Choosing, Deciding, or Participating: What Do Patients Want in Primary Care? *Br J Gen Pract* 2008;58(554):603–604. https://doi.org/10.3399/bjgp08X330681

2. Evans WRH. Imran Rafi, Rare Diseases in General Practice: Recognising the Zebras among the Horses. *Br J Gen Pract* 2016;66(652):550–551. https://doi.org/10.3399/bjgp16X687625

3. Scott K. Adverse Childhood Experiences. *InnovAiT*. 2021;14(1):6–11. https://doi.org/10.1177/1755738020964498

4. Johnson M, Doherty M. Sebastian CK Shaw, Overcoming Barriers to Autistic Health Care: Towards Autism-friendly Practices. *Br J Gen Pract* 2022;72(719):255–256. https://doi.org/10.3399/bjgp22X719513

5. Zucco GM, Doty RL. Multiple Chemical Sensitivity. *Brain Sci* 2021 Dec 29;12(1):46. https://doi.org/10.3390/brainsci12010046. PMID: 35053790; PMCID: PMC8773480

6. Rocque R, Leanza Y. A Systematic Review of Patients' Experiences in Communicating with Primary Care Physicians: Intercultural Encounters and a Balance between Vulnerability and Integrity. *PLoS ONE* 2015;10(10):e0139577. https://doi.org/10.1371/journal.pone.0139577

7. de Mul Jos. Horizons of Hermeneutics: Intercultural Hermeneutics in a Globalizing World. *Front Philos China* 2011;6(3):629–656. https://doi.org/10.1007/s11466-011-0159-x

Ripples on a Pond*

If it is difficult to agree what exactly we mean by health, it is perhaps unsurprising that we also approach *unhealth* in a number of different ways. In both cases, we consider sometimes what is visible through the lens of a microscope, sometimes what patients tell us of their experience, and sometimes other things again. In the many current and past examples of divergent behaviour, ability or identity which have fallen under the medical gaze, we examine society's attitude to a person, and the various restrictions, freedoms and obligations which this confers on them. The spectrum of unhealth therefore stretches from the scientifically concrete, a bacillus of *Mycobacterium leprae* stained red on a glass slide, to the socially metaphorical, a leper exiled from their former life and separated by water from family and friends.[1]

We can think about how these things fit together. If *disease* is like a stone dropped into the pond of someone's life, *illness* and *sickness* are concentric ripples representing its effect on them personally and in their wider interactions with people around them.[2, 3] We might add another, *burden*, reflecting the impact of their condition on the smooth running of the health service. Patients and doctors generally find it easiest to talk about disease, the most easily grasped, and a convenient synecdoche that includes the others. Dealing with a disease generally addresses the corresponding illness, sickness and burden, in which case it isn't really necessary to distinguish between them.

There are other circumstances, though, in which this is less clearly so. It is possible to have a disease identified at an early stage without any corresponding illness, although it may still cause sickness if treatment or

* An earlier version of this piece was published as: Hoban B. Ripples on a pond. *Br J Gen Pract*. 2025 Mar 27;75(753):171. doi: 10.3399/bjgp25X741201. PMID: 40147968; PMCID: PMC11961170.

DOI: 10.1201/9781003652045-50

monitoring necessitate time off work, as well as a certain burden. Illness without disease can be hugely problematic for patients, who know there's something wrong and understandably seek the validation of a clear cause, and for doctors, who try to take hold of a solid diagnosis, only to feel it slip through their fingers like fine mud at the bottom of the pond. Sickness can exist in isolation too: a person may be legitimately signed off work because of circumstances which make their job impossible, even if their illness only exists within this unhealthy situation, and the NHS carries no burden as a result. Similarly, most patients taking cholesterol-lowering medication for primary prevention are neither diseased, nor ill, nor sick, although they have been identified as potentially burdensome, a risk to the system which must be mitigated. In each of these cases, we are dealing with circles which overlap to a greater or lesser extent, or sometimes not at all. How they relate to each other is less clear; they certainly no longer conform to the picture of tidily concentric ripples.

There is a hierarchy in unhealth too, in which the objectively verifiable ranks above the subjective, just as psychological conditions come below physical ones. In this context, disease connotes genuineness: however real someone's illness, there is still on both sides of the consultation a preference for framing it in ways that feel unambiguous.[4] We can see this bias reproduced in screening programmes, which aim to uncouple the cure of disease from the treatment of illness, the tidy from the messy.

Our default approach in any consultation is to observe the ripples on a patient's pond so that we can reach into the water and find a stone, and this works often enough that when our first attempts fail, we usually just try harder. Ripples can also be caused by a passing breeze, though, or by the normal activity of fish; they may even be due entirely to our own efforts as we grope around for stones on the bottom. The reality is that ponds are not sterile containers of water patiently waiting for someone to lob things into them, and nor for most people is life a straightforward business interrupted only by disease. In order to interpret a pattern of disturbances on the surface of either medium, we need to have a better understanding of the medium itself and the whole range of ways in which it is disturbed. In truth, we stand at the edge of an ocean rather than a pond, and if we think only in terms of treating diseases, and simply extend into the deeper water the techniques that work well in the shallows, we will drown. And yet, the deeps are where the majority of life takes place, and where patients find themselves in difficulties most often.

Just as it is reasonable to conceive of health in different ways, it is essential if we are to help our patients that we also recognise and address the corresponding modes of unhealth. When there is a clear disease, it requires little imagination to treat it. When we are confronted with illness, however, we must also be able to see the individual; with sickness, society; and with burden, how the individual relates to the system. Health is regularly diminished by many things and in many ways, and our approach as doctors should reflect this. We all reach instinctively for the microscope, but if we can distinguish more clearly the context in which people who are unwell consult us, we may find that we are often in a position to do less and achieve more.

References

1. Sontag Susan, *Illness as Metaphor*. 1st ed. Farrar, Straus & Giroux, New York, 1978.

2. Helman C. Disease versus Illness in General Practice. *J R Coll Gen Pract* 1981;31:548–552.

3. Marinker M. Why Make People Patients? *J Med Ethics* 1975;I:81–84.

4. Schone Harry Quinn, *Contested Illness in Context: An Interdisciplinary Study in Disease Definition*. Routledge, Abingdon and New York, 2019.

Having Mental Health

There is something odd about the way in which we have come to talk about emotional or psychological problems. It has become normal to refer to *having mental health* as if this were somehow a bad thing. Naturally, we mean a mental health problem, and I don't mean to be pedantic, but have you ever heard anyone refer in the same way to their physical health? We are used to talking in detail about our bodies and the various ways in which they let us down, but it's as if we only have a vague sense of how our minds work and don't quite know what to say when something goes wrong. I have been consulted by some patients who seemed genuinely to lack the words to say more than "I feel like shit, doctor," and by others who talk about being depressed, manic, paranoid or psychotic, using these terms loosely in a way that obscures what they are trying to describe.

Similarly, we talk about feeling suicidal as if the word had a fixed and specific meaning. It is certainly meaningful but it must be unpacked carefully, like an abandoned suitcase at a train station, or in layers, like a set of matryoshka dolls. Do you ever feel as if it's getting harder to keep going? Do you sometimes fall asleep thinking you wouldn't mind if you didn't wake up again? Are there times when you wonder what it would take to put an end to it all? Have you looked into it seriously? Do you have the stuff you would need? What's holding you back right now? As with the word *literally*, usage varies.[1] By asking proactively about *suicidality*, we've made it easier to use a word, but harder to know what someone means by it, and perhaps easier to overlook the more subtle indicators of risk. Goodhart's Law states that when a measure becomes a target, it often ceases to be a good measure, and this applies to words as much as statistics.[2]

DOI: 10.1201/9781003652045-51

The way we talk about mental ill health can end up creating a linguistic black box which we see but cannot see inside. How then can we know what to expect from our distressed patients, and how best to help them? Are they well served by medical treatment and the sick role, or should we try to normalise experiences that, to one degree or another, are near-universal?[3] There is a danger that well-intentioned interventions may be counter-productive. The use of trigger warnings, for example, has been shown to increase feelings of anxiety and reinforce the idea that past trauma is central to someone's identity.[4]

Just as pain is an unpleasant sensation that, by and large, helps us to navigate life safely, negative emotions have their place too. Sadness is a healthy reaction to loss, fear to threat or uncertainty, anger to injustice, and disgust to the breaking of social norms. These feelings are all physiological in the sense that despite being uncomfortable, they may be appropriate to our circumstances: they are adaptive, allowing us to attract sympathy and help, or motivating and guiding our actions. Mental illness, by contrast, is pathological in that what we think and feel are incongruent with our situation and have a negative impact on normal function.

Chronic situational stress is commoner than mental illness, although it sometimes leads to it. Our emotional responses may be entirely appropriate, but are nevertheless maladaptive simply because help is unavailable or circumstances are too complex or entrenched for us to be able to change them. Rather than enabling us, our thoughts and feelings wear us down. Stress can be buffered or offset through various coping strategies or forms of support, but the source of the problem is located outside our minds, and simply treating our minds cannot fix it.

These are broad brush-strokes which fail to take into account the nuances of both mental illness and normality, but they are an attempt to move beyond simply "having mental health." Now that we have arrived at a point in our culture where it's considered acceptable to talk about our feelings, it is crucial that we also help our patients find the words with which to express themselves constructively.[5] The great danger otherwise is that we blur too much the boundaries between the physiological and the pathological, between mental illness and situational distress, making it harder to know how we can help. We have already made it the norm for people who wouldn't previously have been considered ill to see themselves in this way, and for this to lead sometimes not to sympathy, understanding or practical support, but rather to medication, personal validation and avoidant behaviour, while those who need our help most have trouble accessing it.[6] Mental health is about more than just feeling happy or avoiding psychological discomfort. It is about being able to see oneself and the world clearly, and thinking, feeling and acting in a way that flows from this.

References

1. Gill Martha, Have we literally broken the English language? *The Guardian*, 13 August 2013. https://www.theguardian.com/commentisfree/2013/aug/13/literally-broken-english-language-definition

2. Wikipedia entry for Goodhart's Law (accessed 4 October 2023).

3. Parsons Talcott, *The Social System*. Free Press, Glencoe, IL, 1951.

4. Jones PJ, Bellet BW, McNally RJ. Helping or Harming? The Effect of Trigger Warnings on Individuals with Trauma Histories. *Clin Psychol Sci* 2020;8(5):905–917. https://doi.org/10.1177/2167702620921341

5. Linehan Marsha, *Skills Training Manual for Treating Borderline Personality Disorder*. Guilford Publications, New York, 1993.

6. Simon AS. Wessely: "Every Time We Have a Mental Health Awareness week My Spirits Sink". *BMJ* 2017; 358:j4305. https://doi.org/10.1136/bmj.j4305

Irresistible and Immovable Values*

What happens when an irresistible force meets an immovable object? As a society, we want to be tough on crime, while also helping people whose variously disadvantaged and dysfunctional backgrounds make them more likely to offend. Similarly, we are waging war on disease and at the same time dealing with the consequences of overdiagnosis and health-related anxiety. We are caught between imperatives which should in theory be complementary, but tend to conflict with each other in practice: fix things, but look after people too.

The debate in the UK about assisted dying has broadened over the years, such that we are now discussing not just the principles involved, but also the practicalities: what would assisted dying look like in the National Health Service, especially in the context of the current attrition of general practice and palliative care services?[1-3] The thread that runs through the debate, however, seems to be a genuine desire on both sides to help people who are suffering, and the conflict between opposing views reflects not a greater or lesser degree of care, but rather the familiar tension between fixing things – dealing definitively with a problem – and looking after people, even though this may leave the problem unresolved.

Our culture places a significant premium on autonomy, the freedom of any individual to determine their own path in life without undue restrictions, even when their decisions seem unwise or detrimental to their own wellbeing. Terminal illness represents a slow bleeding-out of autonomy, a second childhood of dependence on others for the most basic elements of

* An earlier version of this piece was published as: Hoban B. Irresistible and immovable values. *Br J Gen Pract*. 2025 Feb 27;75(752):123. doi: 10.3399/bjgp25X740877. PMID: 40016103; PMCID: PMC11892768.

DOI: 10.1201/9781003652045-52

daily life, and the inability to end such a life at a time and in the manner of one's choosing is perhaps the ultimate marker of this. The prior testimony of many patients who subsequently travelled to other jurisdictions to end their lives legally is that they took the decision to do this not because of the level of their suffering at the time, but because they would otherwise soon have lost the ability to take such action. The preservation of autonomy is our irresistible force.

Although we value autonomy, we also recognise its limits. These are largely determined by the point at which one person's freedom starts to harm or burden other individuals or society as a whole, although at this point the boundary between private and public domains, is often indistinct or contested. Smoking and drinking are legal but restricted, for example, while most other forms of drug use are proscribed. An individual's decision whether or not to be vaccinated against common pathogens affects not just their own risk of infection, but also the level of immunity within a population, and therefore the risk to others; immunisation against COVID-19 was mandatory for health and social care workers during the pandemic, but not for the general public. The restriction of individual liberties for the benefit of society as a whole represents the social contract, which our prevalent norms of behaviour and legislation reflect, and to which all but the most committed hermits are signatories.

Our culture also places significant restrictions on the taking of life, and this is our immovable object. We have done away with capital punishment; revenge killings and vendettas are the preserve of criminal gangs; and even in warfare, we take pains to avoid harm to civilians and unnecessary violence against enemy combatants. Of all forms of killing, however, suicide holds a special horror for us, such that the merest thought of it is for many patients the reason they seek professional help, and its legacy is a distinctive bereavement laced with guilt and regret.

We are by nature social beings, inhabiting a social medium to which we all contribute, and on which we all rely. Regardless of whether we know one another, and however indirectly, I can only be who I am because you are also who you are. We are defined as much by the web of immediate and more distant connections within which we exist as by our personal characteristics, and killing of any kind is therefore not just a negation of the individual, but also of those connections, a tearing of the fabric into which the threads of all our lives are woven.

Is it feasible, then, for the assistance of suicide to be an act of kindness, and for doctors to participate in it? Trying to help someone end their suffering when death is already fast approaching cannot help but seem reasonable when framed in these terms. We should consider, though, that suffering takes place over the whole course of a life rather than exclusively at its end, and that many people have little autonomy at any point in their lives: do the needs of the dying really diverge so far from those of the living that we are warranted in taking such a radically different approach to them? In our shared world, we can never be fully independent of each other, and the consequences of our actions often go further than we realise. Rewriting the social contract to promote the freedom of the private over the social self in terminal illness necessarily affects the equilibrium of society as a whole, as well as the decision-making of other individuals, including those whose freedoms are already limited by disability or adverse circumstances.

The existence of an irresistible force logically excludes the possibility of an immovable object, and vice versa: a single universe cannot contain both. Neither our respect for personal autonomy nor our taboo against killing represent absolute values, although it is clear in the context of assisted dying that we can only uphold one or the other entirely. We are all committed as doctors to relieving suffering, and yet we also accept on a daily basis that there are many things which we cannot fix, not just because we lack the means, but because the harms associated with them sometimes outweigh the benefits. We can nevertheless still look after people, even when they ask us to help them die, and even if we decide that on balance we cannot.

References

1. Lawson E, Papanikitas A. GPs and Assisted Dying. *Br J Gen Pract* 2025. https://doi.org/10.3399/bjgp25X740409

2. Everington SS. The Assisted Dying Debate: Supporting GPs in a Changing Landscape. *Br J Gen Pract* 2024 February 29;74(740):106–107. https://doi.org/10.3399/bjgp24X736485. PMID: 39222413; PMCID: PMC10904124

3. Lamb L. Crossing the Rubicon, Assisted Dying in General Practice. *BJGP Life*, 4 January 2025. https://bjgplife.com/crossing-the-rubicon-assisted-dying-in-general-practice/ (accessed 6 January 2025).

Archery, Noodles, and General Practice

In 1924 a German academic named Eugen Herrigel travelled to Japan to study archery under Awa Kenzo, an instructor regarded by his peers as a maverick, and well removed from the mainstream of historic *kyūdō*. Herrigel was interested in mysticism; Kenzo's ideas evidently appealed to him, and the result was *Zen in the art of archery*, a book which he published in 1948, and which became for many in the West an introduction to Zen Buddhism, leading to the adoption of Japanese archery as a spiritual discipline. The only snag was that what he wrote had little to do with Zen or traditional Japanese archery, although there are now Japanese people learning a pseudo-Japanese practice introduced by a European.[1]

My point isn't about cultural appropriation, but rather that culture is fluid. Appeals to tradition represent a desire to preserve the evanescent, to build a clear narrative that tells us who we are and how we should go about things, even if its historical basis is shaky. We project our thinking onto a suitable object, which becomes for us symbolic of something with which it may have little original connection.[2] Similarly, our preoccupation with authenticity is based on the idea that people and things have an essential nature, a true and stable self which their appearance and behaviour should reflect. While there is clearly truth in this, it is only one half of the picture: how we live also affects what we are, and both inevitably change over time.

General practice is changing in ways that many of us find deeply concerning, and yet, despite our desire to preserve a traditional, authentic model of care, it is perhaps difficult to say exactly what that means. If there ever was a golden age of general practice, I wonder if it represented simply

DOI: 10.1201/9781003652045-53

a moment in medicine's transition from an essentially narrative and supportive paradigm to a more biomedical and therapeutic one, when the two were briefly, tantalisingly in balance. The changes that brought us to that illusory moment are the same changes that have now carried us past it, and we cannot go back. Consider that the argument for continuity of care is consistently framed in terms of numerical outcomes like admissions avoided and years added to life, as if those were the things that mattered most. We are relational beings, and it should be self-evident that care must be relational too: the idea that all our health-related needs can be met solely from within a body of knowledge originating in dissecting rooms and laboratories is frankly bizarre, and yet here we are.

If change is inevitable, then wisdom lies not in resisting, but in guiding it in a sensible direction. At present, however, we are hampered by a lack of answers to several basic questions. What is the optimum practice size that allows staff to work well together and get to know their patients while still providing the necessary variety of services and benefitting from efficiencies of scale? How many clinical sessions should GPs expect to work in order to provide ongoing personal care without sacrificing their own health or a life outside the surgery? How much difference does partnership make? How can we balance the need for care that is responsive in the short term and joined up in the longer term? If there aren't enough doctors, how can we work together with other healthcare professionals in a way that is safe and effective? Are we primarily responsible to the government for optimising the health of the population, or to our patients, for helping them live healthy lives?

Around the same time as Herrigel was developing his ideas about Zen archery, a brand-new Japanese trend was emerging all by itself. *Ramen*, or noodles served in broth with various toppings, developed from Chinese cuisine, fuelled by American wheat imports after the war, as a cheap and filling meal for the masses; it has become an instant classic, capable of accommodating variety and innovation without a loss of identity.[3] Perhaps that is the issue for us: there are many different ways of doing general practice, and we risk jeopardising our professional identity if we tie it too closely to organisational factors which patients or politicians view as peripheral. If we want a way of defining general practice that makes sense to both these groups, we may not need to invoke tradition or answer all the big questions first, but think instead in simpler terms, like ramen: something medical combined with something personal in a familiar setting. Delicious!

References

1. Shōji Y. The Myth of Zen in the Art of Archery. *The Japanese Journal of Religious Studies* 2001;28:1–2.

2. Hobsbawm Eric and Ranger Terence, eds., *The Invention of Tradition*. Cambridge University Press, Cambridge, 1983.

3. von Bremzen Anya, *National Dish: Around the World in Search of Food, History and the Meaning of Home*. Pushkin One, London, 2023.

Narrative Failure

It was a Tuesday, I think. Morning surgery had come and gone with the usual mix of phlegm, tears and frailty, and my last patient was sitting in front of me, like a steely-eyed sentry guarding the road to a hurried lunch-time sandwich. Well then, let's see.

"I can't find the words, doc." He was middle-aged, medium height, a little overweight, with no obvious scars, tattoos or other distinguishing features; casually dressed, nothing that really caught the eye, and only the occasional entry in his notes for low back pain or coughs and colds. He looked frightened.

"Can you give me a smile, please...now lift your arms...super." Not a stroke, then.

"It's like I've lost my voice, could it be a virus?" Nothing wrong with his voice though.

"I'm not myself, but I really can't say who I am..." Sounding a bit more mental-healthy now. I tried to remember if that Primary Care Network thing was still running, or was it only on Wednesdays?

"Why don't you tell me how it all started, and we can go from there?" Nice open question, I told myself. Why isn't there ever a registrar around to be impressed when I get that stuff right?

"That's just it, doc, I can't say! I feel like here I am, and I've got something, but it's all a mystery to me." Something shifted in my head, and I heard the sound of a penny dropping in a bank vault deep underground. I rummaged around in my desk for the Campbell-Frank analyser and applied the scalp electrodes and mask with trembling hands. As I looked at the display, I realised that neither of us had said anything for a while, which kind of made sense. The dramatic axis was indicating non-resolving tension, but with a

DOI: 10.1201/9781003652045-54

trope/antitrope count close to zero and a plot trace that could barely make the effort to flatline: total narrative failure.

People often think of GPs as being a bit wishy-washy. You know the sort of thing; you go in with a chest infection and they want to know how you feel about it. It's a fair cop really, but what they don't get is that actually most of life is like that. It's not just what happens that matters to us, but what it means, how we make sense of it, how it fits into our story. When patients complain, it's not usually because anyone's done anything outrageous, but because the facts end up organising themselves into a narrative with elements like "I kept asking for help" and "No one listened to me." When I was growing up, there was a craze for those choose-your-own-adventure books that let you decide what happens next and turn to page so-and-so; I think there's something similar on Netflix now. It was fun to be the hero in the story, although I had a habit of landing on page whichever-it-was with the words "Your adventure ends here."

"Okay, it looks like there's a problem with your narrative organ. It's actually quite common, and plenty of people have a mild form without ever realising it. Yours is much more severe though, and seems to have come on quite suddenly, which explains why it feels so jarring. It tends to affect people with a very concrete outlook, and there's a strong association with over-reliance on conversational clichés. What's the last thing you can remember doing before you made your appointment?"

"Well, I was on the phone to my brother because he'd had Severe Chest Pain and got Rushed into Hospital in case it was a Massive Heart Attack. It turned out to be a False Alarm, but he told me to Get Checked Out, and Better Safe Than Sorry."

I winced at his relentless capitalisation. "Do you think I need a Scan?"

"Sorry," I replied. "I'm Just a GP, I can't request that, but you can Go Private if you want to." I blamed my own capitalisation on an empty stomach; I could feel myself getting tetchy.

If you want to make better sense of your experience, you need to start connecting things with each other, go from A to B to C and so on. A bit of metaphor usually helps glue the different parts of your story together, if you know what I mean.

Can't you just give me a pill or something? I tried using a metaphor once, but it got wedged.

I'm sorry, I don't think a pill will help, but now that we know what the problem is, there are a couple of other things you could try. I can send you a link to some exercises online and refer you to a narrative therapist, although there is a bit of a waiting list.

Let me just get this straight then, doc: my brother has a close shave with the Grim Reaper, I try to look after myself and do the NHS a favour by making an appointment with you instead of going to A&E, and the best you can come up with is some old rubbish about telling a story?

Yes, that's fantastic! See how well you're doing already? Just keep it up and come back and see me again in a week.

I never did see him again to find out how his story went on, but sometimes it's enough just to know that you've helped someone, right?

PART IV

How We Look after Ourselves and Each Other

Being a GP means working with knowledge, skill, wisdom, professionalism and kindness, all in the context of ongoing relationships with our patients and colleagues. It is both a privilege and a responsibility, and there is usually more to do in a given day than will fit into the time available; even within the same morning or afternoon surgery, we can feel at times buoyed up or worn down. Our role offers us a larger degree of agency than many, although in the face of suffering which we cannot always relieve, demand of one kind or another which seems never-ending, and bureaucracy which ties our shoes together and fills our pockets with lead weights, it regularly feels as if it is still not enough. Working in general practice is not easy.

There is a misconception to which we all fall prey at times: that work, like nuclear waste, is inherently toxic, and that we must protect ourselves by either creating rigid walls around it or cultivating the sort of personal qualities that might make us immune to its harmful rays. The danger in taking this view is that we see the problem only in very narrow terms: doctors are insufficiently resilient and need to go on a course; patients are too demanding and should be kept at arm's length; small practices are inefficient and must merge with others.

Care that is relational rather than transactional can feel more draining because it requires more of us; it requires our humanity. For precisely the same reason, though, it also engages and affirms our humanity and therefore protects us from the gradual attrition of the soul that can hollow out a doctor over the years. The answer is not to wrap a cloth around our heart and bury it in the ground for safekeeping. We cannot work like machines,

DOI: 10.1201/9781003652045-55

but we ought instead to realise our advantage over them and use it. The larger view is that we work in a dysfunctional system, of which we can only ever influence a part. Our choices may be limited, and we cannot fix the system, but we can still choose well.

This is the shortest part of the book, and I wonder whether that reflects another sort of bigger picture: there is no silver bullet, no magical way of making general practice easy. Instead, the better we understand what we do as doctors in terms of our thinking, the system, and the consultation, the more smoothly we can navigate the difficulties inherent in our job, the more satisfying we're likely to find it, and the more use we will be to our patients.

Keeping behind the Curve

What would your dream job look like? It might not be in UK General Practice as it is currently, but how much would need to change before that felt less of a stretch? Work is generally a good thing,[1] and jobs in healthcare have the potential to be more rewarding than most. In practice, though, enough things get in the way that the dream has become one of those recurring ones in which you're going on holiday, but no matter what you do, the suitcase won't quite shut. We regularly face a level of demand which we don't have the resources to meet, carry a high level of responsibility within a system that restricts our agency, and do a lot without often feeling as if we've done much good.

To some extent we can fight these frustrations by working harder, bending the rules, and catching up in our own time, at the expense of our personal lives. When things still feel dicey despite this, though, and when we have to keep it up day after day, it's unsurprising when we end up feeling tired, resentful and just a little less human, and the day's patients start to look like the next wave of zombies massing outside the gates. We gradually downgrade our aspiration from thriving to functioning to surviving, and our only options look like pushing through or getting out.

Figure 52.1 illustrates this: it is a crude approximation of the relationship between demand and response in a number of systems, which in our case equate with, respectively, expectation and achievement. Up to a point (1), we simply do more as more is expected of us. Past this point, however, we can go the extra mile but achieve only a little more. When we are already doing all we can (2) but expectations continue to increase, we quickly become less effective. Significantly, the point of maximal achievement (2) is right next to that of system failure (3). Experience suggests that General

DOI: 10.1201/9781003652045-56

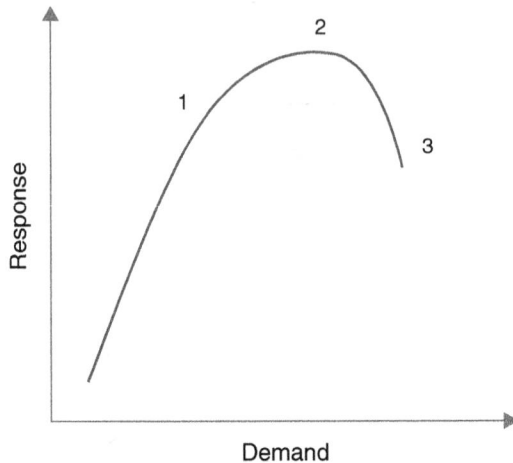

Figure 52.1 Idealised demand/response curve based on a mechanical stress/strain curve, the Frank–Starling Left Ventricular End-Diastolic Pressure/Stroke Volume curve, and the Yerkes–Dodson arousal/performance curve

Practice, the NHS as a whole, and a growing number of individual doctors are all moving from point 2 to point 3. The idea of pushing through has a certain heroic appeal despite being clearly doomed, perhaps only because, like Macbeth, we don't have the energy to do anything else.[2]

We know that a number of personal characteristics are associated with resilience among primary healthcare professionals; it may even be possible to inculcate them through training.[3-5] The danger of seeing this as a solution, though, is that it misses several crucial points.

Firstly, the qualities of resilient doctors are simply those conducive to reasonable psychological health in general,[6] and the majority of people already cope well with any difficulties in their lives.[7] Secondly, most of the variation in individual responses to adversity cannot be accounted for by the presence or absence of "resilience" traits.[8] At best, promoting particular behaviours or attitudes might allow us to adjust marginally the position of transition points on our curve, but its shape and our place on it would remain the same.

Thirdly, and most importantly, resilience is about responding adaptively to crises, not sustaining an unrealistic workload indefinitely. On the graph, it is this adaptability that give us the wiggle-room to stretch from 1 to 2 when we have to, but 1 represents the highest level of demand that can be maintained on a regular basis without damaging the system. If we need to be creative, solution-focussed and hopeful just to make it to the end of an average day, there's something seriously wrong at a higher level than our personal coping skills. There is a danger that we normalise and even celebrate the ability to tolerate chronically and inappropriately high expectations, when we should instead be challenging them.

Look again at the steep slope between 2 and 3 on the graph, though: even a small reduction in demand can quickly improve matters. In other words, if you want to achieve more at this point, take off some of the pressure! In order to be working sustainably, though, we need to push expectations back further, from 2 to 1. In terms of appointments per day, or documents filed, this would mean achieving less, but it would give us back the flexibility to respond to peaks in demand, and finally allow us to shut the suitcase, to work at a pace that is more satisfying because it achieves something meaningful for our patients.

For individual GPs, the most adaptive response to an unmanageable workload may be to get out while you can. All work is not toxic, though, and it may also be that relatively small changes in our expectations, or indeed those of our masters, would allow many of us to work more effectively and enjoyably, to remember our own humanity and that of our patients. Simply going on as we are means marching into oblivion. If instead we want to thrive in practice, we need to find a way of keeping behind the curve rather than ahead of it.

References

1. Csikszentmihalyi Mihaly, *Flow: The Psychology of Happiness*. Rider, London, 2002.

2. *Macbeth*, Act 3, Scene 4: "I am in blood/Stepped in so far that should I wade no more,/ Returning were as tedious as go o'er."

3. Robertson HD, Elliott AM, Burton C, Iversen L, Murchie P, Porteous T, Matheson C. Resilience of Primary Healthcare Professionals: A Systematic Review. *Br J Gen Pract* 2016. https://doi.org/10.3399/bjgp16X685261

4. Eley E, Jackson B, Burton C, Walton E. Professional Resilience in GPs Working in Areas of Socioeconomic Deprivation: A Qualitative Study in Primary Care. *Br J Gen Pract* 2018. https://doi.org/10.3399/bjgp18X699401

5. Matheson C, Robertson HD, Elliott AM, Iversen L, Murchie P. Resilience of Primary Healthcare Professionals Working in Challenging Environments: A Focus Group Study. *Br J Gen Pract* 2016. https://doi.org/10.3399/bjgp16X685285

6. Eley DS, Cloninger CR, Walters L, Laurence C, Synott R, Wilkinson D, The Relationship between Resilience and Personality Traits in Doctors: Implications for Enhancing Wellbeing. *Peer J* 2013. https://doi.org/10.7717/peerj.216

7. Bonanno George, *The End of Trauma: How the New Science of Resilience is Changing the Way We Think About PTSD*. Basic Books, New York, 2021.

8. Martin L, McDowall A. The Professional Resilience of Mid-career GPs in the UK: A Qualitative Study. *Br J Gen Pract* 2021. https://doi.org/10.3399/BJGP.2021.0230

Rethinking Continuity

Life is change, and the same current that brought our profession where it is today will most likely carry us somewhere else tomorrow. The recent focus on continuity of care is welcome in that it demonstrates the positive evidence base for what has always been a central part of our role. If we look at continuity without considering the wider context of general practice, however, we may find ourselves being swept out to sea as we gaze longingly back at the beach.

The context here is that a patient's care over the course of their lifetime now necessarily involves more people than before, as GPs work fewer clinical sessions and change their job more often,[1] other healthcare professionals take on traditionally medical roles, practices become larger and the pressures in the system keep rising.[2] How could it not become more difficult for someone wanting an appointment always to see the same named doctor?[3] It is worth considering too that patients don't always get on with their nominal GP, and would sometimes prefer to see someone else.[4,5] Given the relational foundation of general practice, it would be remarkable if all doctor–patient pairings were equally harmonious or effective. A certain amount of movement within a practice is to be expected before a patient finds the doctor they can work with best, and the danger of trying too hard to prevent this is that the pursuit of continuity ends up becoming a barrier to good care.

The focus on personal rather than organisational continuity also means that we tend to neglect what happens outside our consulting room, when by the time a patient sits down with us, they will probably already have spoken to several of our colleagues, whether receptionists, doctors or other clinicians, all of whom will have formed an impression of them and their

DOI: 10.1201/9781003652045-57

situation. Only a small part of this will ever make it into the medical record, but imagine if we could integrate these impressions with our own: we would not just be better informed, but also have a broader view, based on a number of different perspectives. Where it happens, this integration takes place in clinical meetings as well as less formal professional encounters, circumstances allowing, around the kettle, in the office, or at reception.

Although it's become commonplace to refer to any organisation as a team, it's worth asking how accurate this is. Players in a team carry out their individual roles in a way that is mutually enabling in pursuit of a common objective. Sitting in our room doing our thing while everyone else is sat in their room doing theirs is not teamwork, and yet this is often what happens, especially when it's busy. Chatting with the receptionist over a cup of tea or setting aside time at the end of surgery for clinicians to discuss cases can feel like a luxury, but I would argue that they're actually vital to ensuring that we function as a team, and that losing these moments of interaction makes us less effective and less resilient. There's been a healthy shift in professional thinking from push-through-or-burn-out-trying to look-after-yourself-to-look-after-your-patients, but we may need to widen our perspective to include our colleagues too. The danger of thinking just about how we can protect our own wellbeing is that it quickly turns into a zero-sum game or a race to the exit. The bigger picture is that by working well together and looking after each other, we will find that we are also taking better care of ourselves and our patients.

It's easy to think of continuity as a treasure chest buried on the desert island we have left behind us, which we must choose either to abandon forever or recover at any cost, but this is a false dichotomy. The current is carrying us forwards, and by allowing ourselves to follow it, we have the chance to move towards a richer kind of continuity based not on the contributions of just one individual, but on those of the whole team. We have always acknowledged the importance of the doctor–patient relationship, but by looking at the relationship between patients and the practice as a whole – and the relationships within the practice – we can ensure that in a changing healthcare context, continuity of care becomes multifaceted rather than fragmented.

References

1. Parisi R, Lau Y, Bower P, et al. Rates of Turnover Among General Practitioners: A Retrospective Study of all English General Practices between 2007 and 2019 *BMJ Open* 2021;11:e049827. https://doi.org/10.1136/bmjopen-2021-049827

2. NHS Digital, General Practice Trends in the UK to 2017 Technical Steering Committee (TSC) Archive – NHS Digital. https://digital.nhs.uk/data-and-information/areas-of-interest/workforce/technical-steering-committee-tsc/technical-steering-committee-tsc-archive

3. Tammes P, Morris RW, Murphy M, Salisbury C. Is Continuity of Primary Care Declining in England? Practice-level Longitudinal Study from 2012 to 2017. *Br J Gen Pract* 2021;71(707):e432–e440. https://doi.org/10.3399/BJGP.2020.0935

4. Changing Doctors without Changing Address. *J R Coll Gen Pract* 1986;36(285):185. https://bjgp.org/content/bjgp/36/285/185.full.pdf

5. Billinghurst B, Whitfield M. Why Do Patients Change their General Practitioner? A Postal Questionnaire Study of Patients in Avon. *Br J Gen Pract* 1993;43(373):336–338.

Professionalism, Kindness, and Going the Extra Mile

The General Medical Council (GMC)'s requirement in its updated guidance *Good Medical Practice* for doctors to be kind has caused some consternation.[1] Although it seems reasonable at first glance, the idea that proper medical treatment is dependent on our kindness attributes more agency – and therefore responsibility – to individual practitioners than most of us would own, and seems likely to feed into the blame culture of the NHS.[2] The perception that someone has been unkind is already a frequent trigger of complaints, and in situations where we have a responsibility to challenge patients, should we instead just avoid rocking the boat? Is this really kindness? The GMC is the arbiter of professionalism in medicine, but how does being kind fit into a professional framework, and is it a luxury or a necessity?

Professionalism is partly about training, competence and conformity to accepted standards of practice. What really defines us as professionals, though, is that the role becomes part of our identity: we don't just *do medicine*; we *are doctors*. This means that we have a degree of autonomy in how we practise, but only within our wider responsibility to know the rules of the game and play by them. If we don't wear a uniform, it's not that we have cast it off, but that we have internalised it. We are less free than we appear.

When patients and doctors look at each other, they see not just the *other*, but a person like themselves, and it is this sense of shared humanity, of kinship, that is the basis for effective relationships within which kindness finds its place.[3] The patient says, in effect, "Please help me because I am like you," and we act professionally on their behalf, not just because it is our job, but because we recognise the validity of their appeal. Our shared humanity motivates us to help, and our professionalism defines the help we offer.

DOI: 10.1201/9781003652045-58

Recognising and preserving the distinction between professionalism and humanity in our relationships is crucial. Otherwise, a patient asking for something that their doctor cannot reasonably give may misinterpret refusal as a denial of kinship and take offence. Conversely, a doctor seeking to affirm the same sense of kinship may end up over-sharing or prescribing inappropriately. If there is a causal link between burnout and the over-prescribing of antibiotics and opioids,[4] might this represent not so much a professional failure to say no as an aching human need to say yes – to try, however clumsily, to introduce some kindness into what can easily become a dehumanising experience of work?

There is in each of us a need to be kind, to use the resources at our disposal in a way that sustains positive relationships with those around us, whether colleagues or patients. And yet, if we constantly go the extra mile and give more of our time, attention and energy, there is a danger that we end up either exhausting ourselves or trying so hard to avoid exhaustion that we lock away our humanity behind a professional façade.[5] The problem is, in fact, neither an excess nor a lack of kindness, but a misunderstanding of the role of kindness in professional relationships.

It is perhaps worth reflecting on the origin of the metaphor of going the extra mile. A first-century Roman soldier could require a local to carry his gear for one mile, after which he was freed from further obligation, but Jesus told his followers to double this distance.[6] He wasn't supporting the military, but subverting the paradigm of power and control. True strength is about more, and kindness need not weaken us.

In motivating us to do what we can, then, kindness does often lead us to go beyond the bare minimum. This is not just a zero-sum transaction in which we deplete ourselves for our patients' benefit, however. Rather, by affirming and strengthening our kinship, it lets us build relationships in which patients are willing to take on greater responsibility for their own healthcare, share more of the uncertainty that is ever-present in medicine, and forgive us more readily when we get things wrong. Kindness is neither a luxury nor an obligation, but a fundamental part of how we relate to each other. Put simply, we cannot afford not to be kind, especially when we are busy.[7]

The inclusion of kindness in Good Medical Practice is, on the face of it, a reasonable reflection of the importance of relationships in medicine. In locating kindness within the professional rather than the human sphere, however, the GMC has made a category error with serious implications. Good doctors will always go the extra mile, but, by definition, this is not something that can be required of them.[8] There is a danger that kindness, like resilience or continuity, becomes just another magical solution to the problems of the health service, when what we really need is a system in which a doctor's kindness unlocks the appropriate professional resources, rather than creating an obligation to make up for their absence.

References

1. McCartney M. The Job of a Doctor is Not Necessarily to Be Kind. *BMJ* 2023;382:p1995. https://doi.org/10.1136/bmj.p1995

2. From a blame culture to a learning culture: Health Secretary addresses the Global Patient Safety Summit on improving safety standards in. https://www.gov.uk/government/speeches/from-a-blame-culture-to-a-learning-culture

3. Ballatt J, Campling P. *Intelligent Kindness: Reforming the Culture of Healthcare.* RCPsych Publications, 2011.

4. Hodkinson A, Zghebi SS, Kontopantelis E, Grigoroglou C, Ashcroft DM, Hann M, Chew-Graham CA, Payne RA, Little P, de Lusignan S, Zhou A, Esmail A, Panagioti M. Association of Strong Opioids and Antibiotics Prescribing with GP Burnout: A Retrospective Cross-sectional Study. *BJGP* 2023;73(733):e634–e643. https://doi.org/10.3399/BJGP.2022.0394

5. Stone L. Rationing the Milk of Human Kindness: The Fable of the Dun Cow. *BJGP* 2020;70(698):456. https://doi.org/10.3399/bjgp20X712457

6. The Bible, Matthew 5:41, New International Version.

7. Mathers N. Compassion and the Science of Kindness: Harvard Davis Lecture 2015. *BJGP* 2016;66(648):e525–e527. https://doi.org/10.3399/bjgp16X686041

8. Hewett M. Ethics and Toxic High-workload Work Environments. *BJGP* 2022;72(718):226–227. https://doi.org/10.3399/bjgp22X719333

Being Human

You have to know quite a bit to be a doctor, but it's remarkable how easy it is to feel stupid. Guidance changes constantly based on the latest research, or more often on economic or organisational grounds, and any patient with an internet connection and some time to kill in the waiting room can self-diagnose half-a-dozen conditions you've never even heard of. Wouldn't it be nice to be able to download the latest updates in your sleep and go to work knowing that you were fully NHS-compliant, and without having to dodge any of those awkward questions about Segawa Syndrome? It certainly feels as if you need to be a bit of a machine to keep up sometimes.

The steady flow of extra work from other parts of the system often reinforces this impression, as lists of GP-to-do tasks land on our desk, compiled by someone at another desk juggling their own lists, who either thinks these jobs are necessary but isn't in a position to do them, or is just passing them on from someone else. It can feel at times as if we're stuck inside a vast machine, cogs turned by other cogs, with little real agency; it's just a bit dehumanising.

At the same time as we're trying to make people work like machines, we're also busy trying to make machines more like people. Alan Turing famously proposed the ability to convince a person that they were talking to another person as a test of Artificial Intelligence (AI). This assumes that people think and communicate in typically "human" ways, which machines can learn to imitate, but what if machines and humans are just converging as each tries to imitate the other? Have you ever had trouble online completing a CAPTCHA to prove that you're a real person?

Underlying much of our ambivalence about AI is the suspicion that humanity is simply a function of intelligence, and that intelligence is the

DOI: 10.1201/9781003652045-59

same as whatever computers have that keeps on getting bigger, faster or generally more impressive: at some point we will be left behind. We can accept the idea that a computer is made from microchips containing millions of tiny switches that allow them to store information, but I suspect that for most of us, it's unclear how this allows us to write up our notes, send e-mails or watch videos of kittens on the internet. We default to the analogy that computers are like brains, and it's not a big jump to start giving them names and talking to them as if they were people. *Alexa, think for me.*

Still, few would go so far as to say that intelligence is all it takes to be human. Consider the evil genius character in so many stories, whose humanity seems diminished by an intellect lacking in other human qualities to balance it: computational power alone is not enough, and yet we sometimes hanker after it as if it were. It is not the sentient robots from which we need to be protected, but our own thinking that makes them seem desirable, the fever-dream of perfect solutions implemented by interchangeable drones.

Where does this leave us then, as doctors and as people? We are a mixed bag, fallible and inconsistent, and our fascination with AI has something of the evil genius about it, as if, by force of will, we could remake humanity without its flaws. In fact, we have already gone down this path by basing our healthcare system on knowledge, standardisation, and professionalism at the expense of more meaningful personal interactions. This means, in theory, that we will always get the best treatment for our condition, regardless of who provides it. In practice, however, such a system necessarily privileges the biomedical understanding of ill health and is too intolerant of ambiguity, giving the message that only a person who has been medically investigated and optimised can be said to be healthy. The result is disempowered patients and overloaded doctors. It is a system in which machines could care perfectly for other machines, but one that creates a hostile environment for people on both sides of the desk.

When we feel helpless or overwhelmed by all that we face at work, it is not because we lack the brains to come up with a solution. It is rather that we are being human in a context in which humanity is routinely undervalued, and sometimes there are no solutions. We all need a sense of agency, an understanding that what we're doing is meaningful in a way that goes beyond merely fixing things, and this comes not from perfect knowledge, but from relationships in which both sides extend goodwill to the other and reach an understanding of how to proceed in the face of uncertainty. Our strength lies not just in our intelligence, but also in our other human qualities – and our patients need both. Trying to keep up with the machines is a race we can never win, nor is it one we need enter. Let's keep being human.

Overcoming the Monster

Most of our struggles are mundane, a steady shovelling to clear a path while snow falls from a lowering sky; neither our contract nor our humanity requires us to strap on armour and march, spear in hand, into the lair of some fanged and hairy terror to do battle. There is still a quiet heroism, though, in shovelling, especially as the light starts to fail and wolves roam. Looking after people in general practice often requires a certain heroism too, as paperwork silently accumulates, the list of urgent extras grows, and the risk of a missed diagnosis or complaint bares its teeth. How we understand our story makes a difference to how we go about the job, how effectively we do it, and how it leaves us feeling when we go home. Although the total number of stories must be infinite, most recapitulate a small number of underlying narrative structures and themes, familiar tunes played in a variety of styles. One of these proto-narratives is especially relevant to us as doctors: Overcoming the Monster.[1]

The plot follows a sequence of five stages. First, we are introduced to the immature hero (male or female) and the monster: a dragon, tyrant, or some other undefined dark power. Next, the hero somehow acquires a selection of special abilities, allies or equipment, which seem to guarantee success in dealing with the monster. In the third stage, it soon becomes apparent, however, that the monster is far more powerful than we first realised. Our hero, undaunted, presses on to stage four, in which battle commences, but is soon in serious trouble and about to be defeated. In the final stage, just as disaster seems inevitable, the hero gains some kind of last-minute advantage, snatching victory from the jaws of defeat.

Naturally, good must triumph over evil, and yet there is little dramatic tension when the outcome of any fight is a foregone conclusion. The hero's

DOI: 10.1201/9781003652045-60

advantage, therefore, never lies simply in being stronger than the monster, but in using something other than strength: insight in finding a weakness to exploit; a willingness to pursue the more uncertain course of action because it feels right; or the ability to enlist the help of others. However powerful the hero, the monster is, by definition, more powerful, and so it is only by approaching things differently that the hero can defeat it. The subtext is that we mature not just through mastering our existing capabilities, but through balancing them with complementary ones: strength with skill; knowledge with wisdom; competence with care.

If we consider how this might apply to our work as doctors, the reality is that all too often, we undervalue what seem like the softer elements of these pairings. We often distrust fast, intuitive thinking, for example, preferring to reason things out slowly, logically, so that we can see our own workings.[2] We privilege values such as objectivity, consistency and autonomy, but often overlook others like responsiveness, connectedness, and sensitivity to context.[3] The motto of the Royal College of General Practitioners may be *Cum Scientia Caritas*, but Scientia usually seems to win. These splits reflect dual aspects of how our minds work, and of who we are: we lean into the world with one, experiencing and engaging, and lean back from it with the other, dissecting our experience and reconstructing the abstract concepts and narratives with which to make sense of it.[4] We cannot manage with only half a soul, however hypertrophied; it should be obvious that we need both.

When we talk about general practice as "the integrating discipline," we tend to mean that it integrates the different parts of our patients and their care.[5] I would argue that the term applies equally to the integration of these complementary aspects of what we do as GPs, and perhaps also to the integration of different ways of working within a practice: one of the distinctive features of any band of heroes is its diversity; the uniform and faceless stormtroopers are always the bad guys. There is a great danger that as our workload continues to rise, we respond simply by working harder, faster and in ways that are more focussed but also narrower, and ultimately less intelligent, less caring and less effective.[6] We are summoning up all our available strength to overcome the monster, and we are struggling. Is it possible that we need not just more strength, or more doctors, but also a renewed focus on the complementarity that makes us distinctive? We cannot keep absorbing more work indefinitely, but by choosing to build strong relationships within our practices, by giving patients the confidence to look after themselves better, and by rejecting the creeping "taskification" of what we do,[7] we may yet be able to snatch victory from the jaws of defeat ourselves.

References

1. Booker Christopher, *The Seven Basic Plots: Why We Tell Stories*. Bloomsbury, London, 2004.

2. Kahneman Daniel, *Thinking, Fast and Slow*. Penguin, New York, 2012.

3. Baggini Julian, *How the World Thinks: A Global History of Philosophy*. Granta, London, 2018.

4. McGilchrist Iain, *The Master and his Emissary: The divided brain and the Making of the Western Mind*. 1st edition. Yale University Press, New Haven, CT, 2009.

5. Gray DP. General Practice – The Integrating Discipline. *Br J Gen Pract* 2023;73(734):388–390. https://doi.org/10.3399/bjgp23X734697

6. Mullainathan Sendhil, Shafir Eldar, *Scarcity: The True Cost of Not Having Enough*. Penguin, New York, 2014.

7. Khan N. Are We Seeing More Complex Patients and, If So, Why? *Br J Gen Pract* 2024;74(741):177–178. https://doi.org/10.3399/bjgp24X736929

Making It Look Easy

Bosco hit the ground running, literally. Transport would be well clear of the drop zone by now, and with Control offline until 0800, she was on her own. The Clinical Director's flash transmission had sounded routine, but she could feel that something was off even before she made the suit with the newspaper coming round the fountain in the middle of the square; by the time he unholstered his Glock, she'd already cleared the picnic table he was banking on to slow her down, and was coming out of the monkey vault and considering her next move, pleased that she'd picked up the jacket with the extra elastane in the sales. She was unarmed, didn't want any extra weight to slow her down, but this neighbourhood was her playground, and she already had the advantage. The drop wasn't scheduled for another two minutes, leaving her time to look around and see who else would be joining the party. The nanny with the empty pram at the northeast corner of the square was a bit obvious, as was her partner on the bench, making eye-contact with her every time he sipped his take-away coffee; neither of them seemed to have noticed newspaper guy, or the suspiciously buff crew in fluorescent orange overalls getting out of a utility company van, who looked like they spent more time in the gym than digging holes. Bosco smiled as she vaulted the handrail to the underpass: this was going to be fun.

What most people don't realise is that none of this stuff is difficult if you keep in shape and know what you're doing. To do it well, though, to make it really flow, you have to love it. Bosco felt like she had been running her whole life, one way or another, and you might just as well have asked her to stop breathing as stand still; for her, movement was life. The Primary Care Network job wasn't something she'd really planned, but it had

DOI: 10.1201/9781003652045-61

presented itself at a time when she was looking for a change and didn't need management breathing down her neck all the time, and she had known straight away that it suited her perfectly. People were starting to notice her, and it was getting hard to keep a low profile, but she was too good at it to stop, and she didn't plan to.

The courier entered the south-west corner of the square right on time, looking tense and walking from the direction of the new independent pharmacy, with a plain black nylon satchel over her shoulder. She might as well have been waving a Get-your-controlled-drugs-here sign. Team Orange spread out to form a loose cordon around the fountain, while newspaper guy made a bee-line for the courier, hand sliding under his jacket for some firearm time; she saw him, froze, ditched the satchel and ran straight into the nanny, who'd just emerged from behind an organic juice kiosk, knocking her over and going down hard with the pram. Two of the workmen had newspaper guy pinned down before he could do anything dangerous, while another two scared off the nanny's partner and the last one jogged over to make the pick-up, looking pretty pleased with himself. Bosco came out of the underpass running flat out and totally in the zone, limbs loose and breathing relaxed as she hit the square. Her outfit was a cross between office casual and jogger, and she could see the orange lead hesitate for a second as she closed the distance between them in three fluid strides before dropping into a roll and pushing off with the satchel in her right hand. As he realised his mistake and started after her, he could see that Bosco was headed straight for the fountain and going way too fast to turn around it; instead, she stepped up the side of the parapet, getting a good grip on the brick-work with her trainers, before side-flipping over his head and landing on the balls of her feet in an easy safety tap. He did his best to change direction and catch up, but once she was off, it was straightforward Land Rover-versus-Ferrari.

Bosco had to remind herself to slow down once she'd left the square and disappeared into the back-streets off its south side, knowing that the greater risk now would be attracting attention to herself. She dumped the satchel in a wheelie bin after checking its contents and transferring them to her inside jacket pocket, and settled into a standard commuter gait, walking with shoulders forward and eyes on the ground before turning a corner and approaching Central's main entrance, where a crowd at reception provided natural cover. There was no rush now, and she let the Brownian motion of bodies move her into the building before peeling off and heading for a door marked Staff Only. She opened it using a swipe card with a photo that might have been hers, and a name and job title which she'd made her own: Julie Bosco, Clinical Pharmacist. Control was upstairs in the kitchen, talking in a low voice with the Clinical Director; they both looked up expectantly when she walked in. "Relax, I made the pick-up. You can tell Mrs Jones we've got Billy's Methylphenidate." Relieved smiles all round. "Thanks, Julie, you make it look easy."

Pulp Fiction

Resilience or Something Else?*

I don't know what it was in the end, but something in me just snapped. I needed a fix, although I wasn't really sure what was broken; I wasn't really sure of much anymore. It had all seemed so clear in the beginning: use the science to help people, to look after them. After twenty years, it felt as if something had gone wrong, and things were about as clear as the row of urine samples on my desk; somehow, the ones wrapped in plastic bags always bother me. A lot of things bother me these days: the letters from specialists I've never heard of about patients I've never seen asking me to prescribe drugs I can't even pronounce; the GANFYDs[1] that don't even seem weird anymore because I've seen them all before. Most of all, though, it's the feeling that I'm just the monkey turning the handle on the organ, hoping that it won't fall off. I'm not sure that's what the monkey's meant to do, but the organ grinder went home long ago.

So anyway, I left by the Covid door[2] under cover of a virtual Primary Care Network meeting, figuring that by the time anyone noticed the urine samples building up at reception I'd be long gone. I'd heard of a guy with the kind of clout I was after. I had to lean on some acquaintances I'd made on the Dark Web while sourcing HRT, and they set up a meet with Fat Tony. The place was in the wrong part of town and my directions had been vague, but I knew instinctively that I'd arrived: years spent picking up subtle cues in consultations have that effect. There was also a sign over the door. I went inside not knowing what to expect; the feeling that I'd been coshed over the back of the head definitely came as a surprise. Still, it

---

* An earlier version of this piece was published as: Hoban B. Pulp fiction, resilience, or something else? *Br J Gen Pract*. 2022 Nov 24;72(725):588. doi: 10.3399/bjgp22X721433. PMID: 36424155; PMCID: PMC9710815.

DOI: 10.1201/9781003652045-62

turned out to be the result of having been coshed over the back of the head rather than a sub-arachnoid haemorrhage, so there are up-sides to any situation. When I regained consciousness I was tied to an office chair, which felt oddly familiar. In the background I could hear the clatter of pans, angry voices and what sounded like Verdi. The man opposite me pushed his plate of spaghetti and meatballs to one side and gave me the look that a snake gives a mouse.

"Please excuse my cousin Vincente, he gets a little over-protective sometimes. *Precautions*, you understand. So, you think you want my help, but I gotta be honest with you, doc, you're better off without it. You think you wanna be *resilient*, but all that means is some wise guy gives you a pair of concrete boots and you ask him for a matching coat. *Che idiota!*"

"But what can I do, Don Antonio? I can't retire, and I've got to find some way of coping with all the work. It's the government, you see, the patients..."

"So it's busy and nobody cares. Whaddya wanna do, grow a beard and make sourdough? Fuhgeddaboudit! Show respect to the people you work with. Treat your patients good, like family, and one day they'll return the favour when you need it, or cut you some slack when things go bad. Nobody wants to be looked after by robo-doc, they just need someone they can trust to have their back when they're sick. Now try some of this Barolo and Vinny will take you home."

The Barolo was incredible, rich tannins with a subtle note of -

Okay, so the wine was drugged. When I woke up I was back at my desk with a sore head and drool on the keyboard. The PCN meeting was still going on, and I remembered that it was on the subject of resilience training. I bailed and went to make a cup of tea for the receptionist. The urine samples were looking a bit clearer already.

Notes

1 Get A Note From Your Doctor, i.e. a frivolous request for medical adjudication of a non-medical issue.
2 A separate door used by patients with symptoms of COVID-19 during the pandemic in order to reduce the risk of infection to others.

Index

For Product Safety Concerns and Information please contact our EU
representative GPSR@taylorandfrancis.com
Taylor & Francis Verlag GmbH, Kaufingerstraße 24, 80331 München, Germany